REFLEXOLOGY
and the Intestinal Link

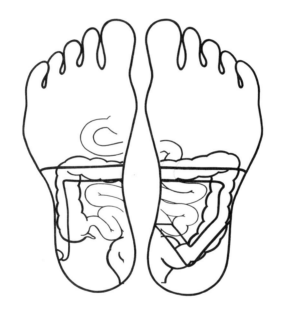

Ann Gillanders

**REFLEXOLOGY
AND THE
INTESTINAL LINK
WALL CHART**
**A coloured Wall Chart
is available to
complement this book.
The Chart enlarges
Diagrams 2 and 3
making the practical
application of the
intestinal links easier
to accomplish.
ISBN 0 9511868 8 4**

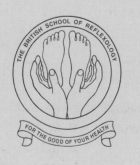

**REFLEXOLOGY AND THE INTESTINAL LINK
by Ann Gillanders**
ISBN 0 9511868 9 2

British Library Cataloguing in Publication Data.
A catalogue record for this book is available from the
British Library.

Text & *Illustrations: Copyright ©Ann Gillanders 1999

Published by Ann Gillanders 1999
Reprinted 2000

Cover and book design by Eleanor Tanner.
Typeset in Palatino by Eleanor Tanner Design,
25 Godfrey Way, Great Dunmow, Essex CM6 2AY.

Printed and bound in Great Britain by The Alden Press,
Oxford.

Acknowledgements: To my great friend Eleanor Tanner, for
the sensitive and artistic design and production of yet another
book - *Reflexology and the Intestinal Link.*

**Illustration copyright acknowledgement:* Most, but not all, of
the anatomy and physiology diagrams are taken from 'The Sourcebook
of Medical Illustration', for which the author has permission: the
copyright is held by The Medical College of St. Bartholomew's
Hospital, London.

All other illustrations including Reflexology diagrams ©Ann
Gillanders 1999.

References: Colon Health by Norman Walker. Published by
Norwalk Press, North Cortez, Suite 2100, Prescott, Arizona.
Understanding Disease by John Ball. Published by Blackdown
Publications, Blackborough, Cullompton, Devon EX15 2HH.

For your information
If bowel abnormalities persist, it is always advisable to consult
a general practitioner.

The Reflexology and the Intestinal Link Wall Chart
and all of Ann Gillanders' books are available direct from
the author: see page 112 for full list and details.

Contents

PART ONE

Introducing the Colon

Continued

PART TWO

Reflexology and the link with the intestinal reflexes

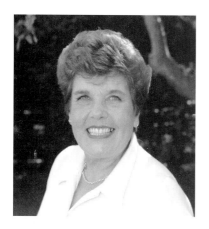

Author profile

ANN GILLANDERS is the Principal of The British School of Reflexology. Ann and her brother Tony Porter were the true pioneers of reflexology some 25 years ago and were responsible for the development of reflexology throughout the United Kingdom. Ann's career has been both extensive and varied, although directed entirely to the fields of medicine and healing.

In 1973 she was introduced to reflexology: at that time it was a completely unknown science, and often ridiculed. Ann trained with Dwight Byers, Director of the International Institute of Reflexology, in Florida U.S.A. After qualifying she established a large practice in Harlow where she still practises today.

In 1979 Ann and Tony undertook a teacher-training course with Dwight Byers and promoted reflexology throughout the United Kingdom side of that Institute, establishing training schools in London, Manchester, Switzerland, Paris and Israel.

In 1986 The British School of Reflexology was founded by Ann Gillanders.

In 1989 Ann studied acupresssure and remedial massage with Dr. Louie Chung, Director of the School of Oriental Medicine and obtained a Diploma in both these sciences.

In September 1997, The British School of Reflexology opened training schools in Hong Kong and Japan.

Ann is now an international author which has led to her success with a reflexology features video filmed in Maui, Hawaii. Ann's publications are listed on page 112.

For further information on these and other mail order products, including books on related subjects, charts and therapy equipment, please contact:

BSR Sales Limited,
The Holistic Healing Centre,
92 Sheering Road, Old Harlow, Essex CM17 0JW.
Telephone 01279 429060 FAX 01279 445234

Reflexology is a science which deals with the principle that there are reflexes in the feet relating to all organs, functions and parts of the human body

Foreword

When the colon is out of balance it is necessary to first clean toxins that have accumulated. We then need to acidify the colon so that acidophilus will be able to establish and grow there.

Your internal bowel health is just like a garden. The soil must be prepared initially so that the seeds can be planted, flourish and grow. In order for healing to take place the environment must be free from toxins and poisons.

I hope that by reading this book you will gain a deeper insight into the workings of the human body, and the link that exists between specific reflex points in the feet with reflex points in the colon, and that by applying the science of Reflexology to these pin-pointed areas, described in detail in Part Two of this book, extra encouragement to heal can be given to this wonderful 'human machine' that has been so perfectly designed with tremendous self healing properties.

I hope also that you will be encouraged to understand and appreciate how disease does begin in the colon and all the healings start there too.

Ann Gillanders

Introduction

Our bowel function is vital to our bodily health. All, yes all, health problems which affect our body originate in the bowel. However, despite the vital importance of proper diet, proper education of the root causes of disease which manifest in this area, and movements of our bowel, the intestinal tract is a taboo subject.

From earliest childhood we are conditioned to regard the movement of our bowels as dirty and disgusting, a habit which we need to get over just as quickly as possible. The whole process is quite an undignified affair, best done in private, and if you are constipated it can be quite a painful event.

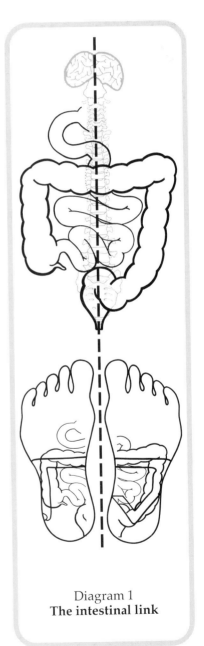

Diagram 1
The intestinal link

PART ONE
Introducing the colon

1 Designed to eliminate – the body's waste disposal unit

The large intestine

The large intestine consists of the colon, rectum and anal canal. The colon begins just above the right groin where it is referred to as the caecum and from which arises the appendix. It ascends on the right side to just below the ribs and crosses over the abdominal area and is, therefore, known as the transverse colon. With a sharp bend called the splenic flexure, it turns downwards and is referred to as the descending colon. The last 'V' bend of the bowel is referred to as the sigmoid colon.

The small intestine

The small bowel is a long and convoluted winding tube leading to the large intestine. The first part, known as the duodenum, is a C-shaped tube 20-25 cm (8-10 in) long. It encircles the pancreas, passes behind the liver in front of the right kidney and across the aorta, the body's largest artery.

The second part of the small intestine is called the jejunum. This is about 2.4 m (8 ft) long and lies in the region just under the navel.

The third part of the small intestine, the ileum, is 3.6 m

(12 ft) long and winds down to the caecum, the first part of the colon or large bowel.

The small intestine is therefore about 6.4 m (21 ft) long and is a good example of compact, accurate design.

Digestion

The surface of the small intestine is an even better example of good design. It has an inner surface area of about 18.6 sq m (200 sq ft) in the average adult and is therefore some ten times larger than the total surface of the skin.

The area is enlarged by millions of tiny finger-like projections called villi, from the Latin word 'villus' meaning 'a tuft of hair', which protrude from the intestinal lining.

Resembling a fine velvet-like carpet, these countless microscopic structures separate valuable particles such as protein, fat and sugar from waste material such as cellulose, an indigestible ingredient and a very rough fibre found in all fruits and vegetables.

Before this happens however, the partly digested food, or chyme, runs the gauntlet of the duodenum where it is bombarded by bile from the liver and digestive juices from the pancreas.

Chyme entering the duodenum from the stomach contains a large proportion of hydrochloric acid which is neutralised by bicarbonate, an alkaline substance, in pancreatic juice. This fluid contains three enzymes, lipase, trypsin, and amylase which break down fats, proteins and starch into respectively small molecules ready for absorption.

The 25 feet of intestinal tubing, is activated by strong peristaltic muscular waves which force our waste products along the bowel to be evacuated at its exit, the rectum.

The remaining tubing absorbs the nutrients from our foodstuffs and distributes these essentials back into our blood stream.

Death begins in the colon... and so do all the cures!

Constipation and diarrhoea

Most people, even children, living in today's modern society are constipated, whether they know it or not. Even people with chronic diarrhoea suffer from one form of constipation.

Chronic diarrhoea is most often due to the presence of irritation in the colon, and/or a stagnant condition of the bowel which is laden with harmful bacteria and even parasites – just the perfect breeding ground for disease to manifest.

Chronic diarrhoea will often respond admirably to a colon cleansing programme which I will deal with later on in this book.

The meaning of the word constipate, has its root in the Latin word 'constipare' which means to press together. Old faeces may build up in pockets and they may coat the entire length of the colon and small intestine as well, so the waste matter becomes hardened and does not become eliminated in normal bowel actions. It is this layer of hardened impacted faeces that causes diseases – diseases of all manner and type.

Apart from the diseases which can manifest from a toxic bowel, an overstretched and laden bowel can descend low into the pelvic cavity and cause pressure on the bladder, rectum and uterus. Many causes of a prolapse of any of these organs can have its origins in the bowel.

A badly enlarged ballooned colon can create excess pressure within the abdomen so that part of the gastro-intestinal tract protrudes through its normal location within the abdominal wall. We refer to this protrusion as a hernia.

If you suffer a hiatus hernia, the stomach protrudes up through an opening in the diaphragm. An inguinal hernia can be seen as a lump in the groin.

By removing the pressure in the colon and cleansing the area it becomes possible for the body to heal itself.

A collapsed colon creates a lack of muscle tone in the

Encourage the body to heal itself

bowel wall, waste products are therefore not activated along the intestinal pathways. The longer food remains in the bowel in a putrefied state the more toxins remain in the system. It is an overload of toxic waste that causes diseases.

The muscles of the bowel are busy all the time, every few seconds they contract briefly: these contractions make the bowel narrower and drive its contents into neighbouring sections which are relaxed.

Most people claim that they open their bowels once a day. The most sensitive time of the day for the bowel to activate is immediately upon waking. Actually getting up from your bed sends a message to the colon to increase the muscular activity. Receiving food and drink sends another important message and that is why breakfast is the most important meal of the day; not only are we breaking-the-fast of the night, but we are also encouraging the evacuation of our bowels.

Inactivity, such as a period in bed because of illness or injury, decreases the muscular contractions of the bowel and we become constipated The elderly who become less active with the normal ageing process also become more prone to constipation.

If constipation is a problem, try to increase your exercise: brisk walking, swimming too is excellent as it exercises the whole of the pelvic area.

Breakfast is the most important meal of the day

The role of bacteria

A unique feature of the large intestine is that it contains a huge number of bacteria which are nearly all harmless. Some animals, the herbivores, depend for their lives on the bacteria in their intestines: the grass they eat is useless until it has been fermented by bacteria.

The bacteria are scavengers living off the undigested remnants of our food, dead cells and the mucus which is produced in the intestine.

It is known that if animals do not have bacteria in their

gut they are more prone to disease.

The average passage time of undigested food remaining in the intestine is about 50 hours. As well as undigested food a stool usually contains a majority of water and a large proportion of bacteria – some living, some dead.

What causes offensive stools and putrefaction of the bowels? What you eat is one cause; the amount of time waste matter remains in the bowel is another. It is possible for food to pass completely through the bowel without putrefying whatsoever. A 100 per cent raw fruit diet gives a non offensive stool, and it is a great way to cleanse the bowel; a raw vegetable diet gives the same result. It is better not to mix fruit and vegetables together if you are trying to detoxify your body.

Body odour

Body odour and foul smelling feet can indicate a toxic colon and putrefaction of the intestinal tract. Overall body perspiration with the exception of underarm perspiration should not create a body odour problem.

The person who has a problem controlling body odour after a normal day's work, and who baths or showers regularly, should consider that their toxic levels are probably on the high side.

High toxic levels indicated

Verrucae

This painful condition which forms as small wart-like growths on the feet which 'seed' and scatter their contents on the soles of the feet and ultimately cause other painful areas to develop are, we are led to believe, caused by a virus which is often picked up at swimming baths or public places where people are walking about with bare feet.

That may be so, but if your toxic levels are high and your feet are eliminating through perspiration this waste which contains high levels of protein, you have the perfect breeding ground for the virus to thrive and multiply.

The need for an acidic colon

The colon is acidic, the main acid being acetic acid. It is believed that this acidity may be one of the body's defences against bacteria.

Antibiotics, all pain killing drugs and steroids have quite a disastrous effect on the bowel, killing off all the active bacteria which leaves more waste in the bowel which should have been ingested by the active bacteria.

The intestine likes dietary fibre. Its enemy is the white flour pappy foods that we consume in great quantities today: bread, cakes, biscuits, pastry etc. Fibre absorbs water, thus bulking out the intestine and encouraging easy evacuation of waste from our bowels.

We hear of 'friendly bacteria'. These produce lactic acid, acetic acid, digestive enzymes and vitamins. The most well known and important species of lactobacteria are Lactobacillus acidophilus and Bifidobacterium bifidus. The name lactobacteria is derived from 'lacto', meaning milk, because lactobacteria produce lactic acid which was first known as the agent generated during the souring of unpasteurized cows milk. The so-called lactobacteria are abundantly present on every blade of grass as well as on most vegetables and grains. Lactobacteria are in milk because cows eat grass.

> The intestine likes dietary fibre

Flatulence

We suffer flatulence when our digestive systems are working inefficiently; not just the bowel but when the stomach, small intestines, pancreas, liver and gall bladder are not producing the right digestive enzymes or when a duct transporting the digestive enzymes is partially or completely blocked.

An excess of flatulence or gas can cause all manner of unpleasant symptoms if it is not expelled readily; headaches are common, so are skin eruptions, lethargy and aches and pains in our joints.

If you have a healthy functioning colon containing the correct balance of intestinal flora there will be several times as many B vitamins present from a well balanced whole food diet. These include vitamin B12 which is essential for preventing and overcoming pernicious anaemia.

MAYBE ALREADY upon reading this chapter you will begin to realise just how vital our intestinal function, which is the 'body's waste disposal unit', is when we begin to look for an improvement in all manner of chronic and acute health problems.

The lymphatic system

As waste material leaves the body cells, it is carried away by the two circulating body fluids, the blood and the lymph.

Lymphatic vessels are concerned with conveying excess fluid, foreign bodies and other materials from the body's cells dealing with waste and potentially harmful substances. It works very closely with the blood, particularly with the white blood cells which are so necessary to the body's strong defence mechanism. The lymphatic vessels (see diagram) run alongside the body's arteries and veins, collecting surplus fluid from the tissues.

Our heart, which is a very strong muscular pump, delivers blood to all parts of our body by strong muscular contractions. Lymphatic fluid is activated by movement, walking, stretching and general exercise and is why we are all encouraged to move as soon after surgery or after an infectious illness as possible. We need to make sure that the lymphatic fluid does not become stagnant. Stagnation of lymphatic fluid leads to an increased risk of infection, phlebitis, thrombosis, and discourages rapid healing of the body.

Lymphatic fluid, although formed out of blood, contains no red blood cells.

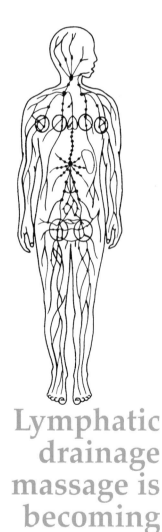

Lymphatic drainage massage is becoming very popular

Every cell in our body, of which we have billions, demands to be bathed in interstitial fluid which consists of materials from our bloodstream together with substances passed out of the cells.

Lymph vessels contain one-way valves and are lined with muscle tissue which pumps lymph through these valves. The lymphatic system's main job is to carry toxins away from all body cells.

Lymphatic drainage massage is becoming a very popular form of massage which is often performed when there is an infection such as flu, bronchitis, etc.

When using lymphatic massage on a sufferer with asthma, sinusitis or bronchitis, the mucus congestion in the body is actually drained into the colon and large quantities of mucus are eliminated through the bowel.

A toxic lymphatic system actually restricts the activity of the white blood cells, so 'if the soil is right, disease will manifest'.

Animals know exactly what to do when an infection invades their bodies, they automatically fast and just drink water – fasting encourages the body to throw off toxins at an increased rate.

When you have a fever, do not eat: most people lose their appetite, that's fine! If you worry that a couple of days on water only will 'be dangerous' disregard this concern and think of the habits of animals, they could teach us many lessons.

...if the soil is right, disease will manifest

Tone up the lymphatic system

To encourage the lymphatic system to work more efficiently, try skin-brushing for about five minutes a day.

Use a firm brush or loofah and with tepid water rigorously scrub your body, starting at the feet and ending at your upper chest and two good herbal lymphatic system purifiers are lobelia and bayberry bark.

PERHAPS WE CAN NOW SEE how inflammatory and congested states occur in the body when the colon is affected, when this happens waste matter backs up into the lymphatic system, and so down we go on the road to disease: toxic waste invades our tissues and disease results.

So again, how vital is our bowel function in regard to health? It is the first step to disease if its abilities are affected by poor diet, insufficient exercise and constipation. Our emotions play a large part in how our bowels behave. Let us look at this now.

2 Mind over matter

Interaction of the mind and bowel

Many of the organs in our body do not give out warning signs when we are under stress: the liver, kidneys and brain, do not consciously vibrate or irritate us when we are in a stressful state. Our hearts, however, beat furiously when we are in an emotional turmoil and we have discomfort in our bladder when we are anxious and need to 'spend a penny' more frequently than usual, but this is easily dealt with.

Our bowels gurgle and rumble, we 'void wind' when stressed and often have to rush to the loo and suffer an embarrassing attack of diarrhoea.

In lay language, stress upsets bowel function which in turn, and in time, allows destructive bacteria in the gut to gain hold and begin breaking down the bowel function. This process can only lead to further disease.

Emotional stress is known to cause alimentary spasm. We quote such phrases in our lives as 'this turns my

Stress upsets bowel function

stomach'; I felt 'sick to the stomach'; 'gnawing fear'; 'butterflies in the stomach'; 'I have a gut reaction' and 'my bowels turned to water'.

The Hara -
the vital centre of man

No function or activity can take place without energy. From the moment of conception, activity is in progress to enable the human foetus to develop. Energy stimulates the glandular secretions, the development of red and white blood cells – in fact every function of our physical body depends on this vital energy – the life force of the human form. Any stagnation results in a decline in energy.

Ancient cultures had a great belief in the link between the psyche and soma (or physical body) and attempted to explain it through reference to the energy systems of the body. We often hear these referred to as the chakras. One of the most important chakras or energy centres is called the Hara or second chakra which is known to control digestion and liver function.

We are encouraged to practice deep, low 'stomach-centred' breathing which is associated with relaxation and response. By simply spending a quiet time each day centring the breathing in this area of the body, we can do much to reduce apprehension and fear.

The solar plexus, which is a complexity of nerves behind the stomach wall, is an area where we hold tension and stress. This area is highly reactive to our emotional state, and a great 'detector' of stress levels in the body, which affect the digestive chakras.

If the colon loses its ability to have a regular and rhythmic peristaltic flow, over a period of time nerve signals stop functioning and large deposits of waste line the muscular wall of the colon, gradually invading the many pockets and convolutions.

This waste paralyses the ileo-caecal valve, backs up into

The Hara or second chakra controls the digestion and liver function

the small intestine and we then have a dangerous toxic condition which is re-absorbed into the blood stream.

Amost every chronic disease known is directly or indirectly due to the influence of bacterial poisons absorbed from the intestines.

These poisons gravitate to weakened spots in the body: maybe an inherited family weakness; an accident resulting in an injury to an organ or structure, i.e. the arthritic hip, spine; or maybe a pattern of childhood illness, such as allergies, asthma, hayfever or stomach upsets.

Even problems with the heart can have a direct association with the alimentary tract.

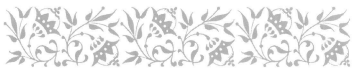

3 Immunity and the colon

Immune responses

It is thought that as much as 80 per cent of immune response is activated from the colon. The colon is well supplied with lymph material in its walls and in the small intestines we have groups of lymphatic cells called Peyers Patches.

There is also a plentiful supply of enzymes in both the colon and the small intestine and these are the immune system's first line of defence.

The appendix too, although considered to have 'no known function', is often referred to as the 'tonsil of the intestine' and is a safety valve for isolating infection, as is the tonsil in the throat, which is a lymphatic gland and is the first line of defence.

80% of immune response is activated from the colon

To remove either the tonsils or appendix without good cause may well drive infection deeper into the body.

Auto-intoxication of the colon

In 1912 this was known and recognized by a group of 57 leading British surgeons who met to look further into bowel hygiene and the increasing problem of auto-intoxication of the colon. Unfortunately all their findings have been ignored and forgotten in the so-called progress of the twentieth century which encourages us to attack all symptoms with drugs, and forget all attempts to treat the root cause of disease.

At that meeting, which was held at the Royal Society of Medicine, it was agreed that their research pinpointed 22 poisons as originating from a toxic colon. These were: phenol, cadaverin, agamatine, indol, sulphuretted hydrogen, cresol, butyric acid, botulin, putrescin, urobilin, histidine, ammonia, muscarine, methymercaptan, indoiam, methygardanine, indoethylamine, sulpherrglobine, ptorrmarropine, penta-methylendiamine, neurin and sepsin.

The decline and fall in education into the function of our bowels and our responsibility for the health of this area throughout the Western World can be directly associated with the increase in degenerative diseases and immune system disorders.

When the immune system of the bowel becomes compromised, extra work is forced on all the remaining systems of elimination.

When the immune system of the bowel becomes compromised, extra work is forced on all remaining systems of elimination

From mother's milk

The first acidophilus implant received is from mother's milk. Nature gives females mammary glands which provide milk (lactol) and bacteria for their young infants' nourishment and immune system.

Mother's milk contains Bifidus, a lactobacteria, and specific growth factors for Bifidus along with important immunoglobulins. These all help establish the basis for a strong immune system in the child. Bifidus constitutes 99 per cent of the nursing infant's colon flora. The presence of this simplified Bifidus flora is considered to be a major factor contributing to the greater resistance to infection and better health of breast fed babies.

The existence of a simplified lactobacteria flora acts as a vital barrier to infections. The colon of the breast fed infant is, by nature, slightly acidic, due to the acid loving and acid secreting Bifidus. This slightly acidified colon prevents the growth of harmful bacteria, which can only thrive in an alkaline environment.

In addition to these acidic secretions, other factors in acidophilus secretions have been found to exert antagonistic actions on the growth of specific harmful types of bacteria. It is primarily due to this action that acidophilus are now generally classified as 'probiotics'.

When the infant begins to eat food other than breast milk, more types of bacteria begin to appear in the colon including L. acidophilus and other beneficial bacteria, along with some harmful types carried on foods of all kinds. This is the change from healthy simplified colon flora of a breast fed infant to a mixed more complex flora.

Healthy colon flora in an adult consists of an estimated 80-85 per cent protective lactobacteria with 15-20 per cent of other types. This balance needs to be maintained through proper diet and lifestyle, to ensure the slightly acidic pH essential for a healthy colon and a strong immune system throughout life.

The bowel of the baby reacts quickly to unfriendly foods and substances: the baby may well have acute attacks of colic, or develop infantile eczema, but as time goes on primary reactions become secondary ones such as severe allergies, asthma, or chronic eczema.

If we simply go about suppressing infantile diseases by

the use of more and more drugs to control symptoms, we are simply forcing disease further and further into the body.

4 Bowel cancer

The statistics

We hear repeatedly about the increase in bowel cancer, indeed 16,000 people die of this disease each year in the UK. Fear then is implanted in our mind when we suffer constipation, pain in the bowel, diarrhoea, or feel bloated and uncomfortable. We fear that maybe our symptoms are of a more sinister origin.

Statistics of bowel cancer are growing and one in twenty people will suffer this disease; women are just as likely to get the disease as men. In fact, cancer of the colon ranks second only to breast cancer and incidents are increasing!

Once again, diet plays a strong part in the development of cancer of the colon. Western diets are high in fats compared to Oriental ones and a twofold difference in colon cancer incidence exists between East and West. Fats have been suspected as the main culprit in the development of bowel cancers and many others.

Can cancer be avoided?

- Eat at least 30 g of fibre a day. High fibre activates the transit time of food travelling through the bowel.
- Increase your consumption of vegetables to at least five servings a day. Higher intakes of vegetables, but not fruit, also seem to have a protective effect.
- Limit red meat intake to one or two servings per week.
- Increase your consumption of fish and fish oils and limit corn oils. Studies in South America have shown that coastal

populations whose stable food is fish have significantly less colorectal cancer.

- Vitamin E is particularly protective.
- Supplement your diet with at least 400mcg of folic acid.
- Take at least 1 gram of vitamin C per day.
- Take rigorous exercise two or three times a week
- If there is a family history of this disease you are obviously more at risk and need to pay attention to all the above recommendations.

The most degrading condition of old age is when we are unable to control our bowel and bladder function, we therefore have an attitude of disgust and embarrassment regarding the function of our bowels.

5 Fear, anger and stress

Affects on the bowel

Fear and anger affects the bowel dramatically and the stress of waiting for the results of an examination can also affect bowel action. Scientists have actually proved that fear can paralyse the low bowel and anger can work it up into excessive activity.

We say we were 'red with anger'; people faint during a stressful situation; our bowels clench themselves during a tense situation; people vomit when subjected to distressing sights such as a road accident. These are all very primitive reactions, but underneath the veneer of living in our civilised society we are all primitive by nature.

In the animal kingdom anger and fear are expressed by roars or screams and fighting releases anger, but in today's world we are expected to hide our feelings. As we hide our feelings from the world, we create stressful feelings in our body which, in particular, affects our bowels. Our gut reactions are totally out of our control.

Considering our ancestors who were hunter-gatherers, when faced with danger defaecation often occurred. This is a response which we must have all experienced. In order to lighten the person in preparation for combat there is a strong desire to open the bowels. Once the bowels were opened, the digestive system shut down until the fighting had subsided. Digesting food was certainly not a necessity in times of crisis.

IBS - Irritable bowel syndrome

Many people in stressful situations suffer from irritable bowel syndrome. This is actually an over sensitive bowel, over sensitive from emotional stimuli and too much adrenaline in the blood stream as the result of anxiety, long term responsibilities – maybe caring for a chronically sick aged parent and fears of any kind that confront us today in this fast paced life.

Women suffer from irritable bowel far more than men who will express their anxieties by developing duodenal or stomach ulcers.

Irritable bowel syndrome was previously known as 'mucus colitis' or 'spastic colon'. Food is said to be responsible for one third of cases but X-ray fails to reveal any specific abnormalities of the bowel. Cows milk and antigens in beef can precipitate the condition.

This chronic condition may cause weight loss and poor health, calling for treatment of the underlying condition. Sufferers are usually hard-striving perfectionists who find it difficult to relax.

The irritable bowel either manifests as chronic episodes of constipation, low pain which usually descends into the left groin, a bloated feeling, excessive wind, or episodes of diarrhoea. The symptoms which are always around lead the sufferer to concentrate on or even to become obsessive about his or her bowel condition which leads to far more irritability. Therefore the mental attitude of the sufferer has a great influence on the severity and duration of the irritable bowel.

Sometimes, escaping from a frustrating relationship which keeps you angry and often depressed is the answer. Other less drastic measures might mean making changes to lifestyle, diet, and learning the ability to truly relax the body, mind and spirit.

6 Balancing the intestinal flora

Host to millions

Human life is only made possible through our co-evolution with the bacterial world. We share an intimate unity with millions upon millions of bacteria which live both in and on us. The place where we house the greatest number of microbes is the intestinal tract. These bacteria and other micro-organisms such as viruses and fungi compose the intestinal flora.

This mass of intestinal flora performs countless functions for the body and is more recently being considered as an organ in its own right.

The bacteria are responsible for numerous metabolic activities, possibly even more than the liver which is noted for its numerous activities. In fact, the liver is often referred to as 'the butler to the brain'!

The state of the intestinal flora is central to health as it is closely linked to the immune function, the detoxification of the body and nutritional status. The quality of our intestinal flora is determined by the balance existing between the various microbial populations. It is

The liver: 'the butler to the brain'

particularly important for a good state of health that the balance between the two predominant groups of bacteria, the Bifidobacteria and the Bacteroides bacteria is maintained.

Due to various degenerative factors affecting our intestinal ecology there is a tendency for the putrefactive Bacteroides bacteria to overgrow. This diminishes the population of Bifidobacteria which can be considered more beneficial to our intestinal ecology.

7 Degenerating intestinal flora

Bacterial malfunction

Lifestyles today are often conducive to forming degenerative intestinal bacteria rather than a flora which supports the healthy functioning of the body. There are various internal and external environmental factors which have a negative effect on the intestinal flora.

One of the main causes of the destruction of this flora is antibiotics: we use antibiotics today far too frequently – babies and children take them from birth, particularly for ear nose and throat infections, bronchitis, etc.

The naturopathic and holistic approach to the causes of respiratory infections consider they arise in the gut and in 95 per cent of cases are due to the inability of the immature digestive system to cope with foodstuffs.

Always remember, babies are born without teeth for a reason, their bodies are not built to cope with a variety of foods until well into their second year when they start to produce large grinding teeth. At this time their digestive systems are mature and able to accept suitable solid foods.

Antibiotics destroy bowel flora

Puppies and kittens are born with a full set of teeth – they need to be independent of their mothers by the age of six weeks – their digestive systems are therefore well able to cope with solid food by the time they are two months old. This is a very different story from the human infant.

Nature has her own time table. If we choose to change the timing to suit ourselves, we will pay the consequences, which are health problems.

Acute infections often become chronic health conditions as the years go by, as we treat, more and more infections with more and more antibiotics.

The frequent throat and ear infections which are treated with ever increading amounts of antibiotics will probably lead to little Johnny having his tonsils and adenoids removed.

The tonsils and adenoids are lymphatic glands, the first line of defence in the body. When these vital glands are removed, it encourages the infection to proceed lower into the respiratory tract.

Repeated attacks of bronchitis and often asthma are the progressive stage of health deterioration, treated with yet more antibiotics, which causes yet more destructive changes in the intestine and consequently more chance of infections.

The intestinal merry-go-round

And so we proceed on the intestinal merry-go-round, never getting very far in our search for improved health and quality of life.

Milk products

Milk products including processed cheeses are the main culprit of causing excessive amounts of mucus production in the body.

Today, as a nation we consume vast quantities of milk products: yogurts, ice creams, milk-shakes, chocolate, cheeses. Our consumption of these foods 40 years or so ago was only on 'high days and holidays' and they were considered to be 'luxury products'.

The medical profession are constantly searching for the elusive 'pot of gold' at the end of the rainbow in their attempts to find the germ or virus that can be blamed for colds and influenza, and more serious diseases. The causes of these conditions are the effects of excessive mucus clogging the body. Eliminate whatever causes the excesses of mucus to form, and infections cannot develop.

A cold is Nature's way of 'house cleaning'. A fever is a 'safety valve'. It is Nature's way of burning up toxic waste that is not being eliminated through the correct channels. When our body is not strong enough to produce a fever to burn up waste, we really do have a problem!

We are what we eat – if we put good performance into our bodies, we can expect good performance out.

The elusive 'pot of gold'

Candida epidemic

The increase in disrupted intestinal ecosystems is leading to problems of bacterial resistance.

We hear so much about Candida albicans which has become a major concern for practitioners in alternative and allopathic medicine.

Candida has become widespread, reaching epidemic proportions. It is an insidious infection which many people have, but are still not aware of it being the root cause of their ill health. This condition can cause much suffering both physically and mentally and is consequently affecting health on a social level.

The Candida species can inhabit virtually every part of the body. There is usually a primary source of infection from which secondary outbreaks of Candida occur. The intestinal tract is most likely the primary site for Candida to reside followed by secondary infections in the mouth, vagina or the nails.

The root like mycelia, which are the tangled mass which make up the feeding and growing part of a fungus, penetrate the gut mucosa, breaking down its function as an effective barrier between the intestinal tract and the rest of the body.

This invasion of the intestinal epithelium increases its permeability, enabling the Candida itself, its toxins, other micro-organisms and waste particles to pass from the intestinal tract into the blood stream. These substances are perceived by the body as foreign particles and therefore evoke an immune reaction.

When these protein particles reach the brain they cause brain allergies which result in a number of personality problems ranging from depression, irritability, sudden mood swings to some schizophrenic symptoms. The constant defensive response of the immune system to the Candida leads to an over-reactive state whereby allergic symptoms occur.

Besides Candida, other micro-organisms such as bacteria, fungi and viruses are able to migrate from the gastro-intestinal tract to other parts of the body causing various inflammatory conditions and infectious diseases. Micro-organisms pass into the lymph nodes, blood and then other organs such as the liver, pancreas and spleen. Bacteria may also adhere to and colonise normally sterile surfaces such as the mucosa of the genito-urinary tract, the lower respiratory tract and sometimes the endothelial surfaces of the cardiovascular system.

It is also common in this condition for the ileo-caecal valve to remain in an open position. This enables colonic bacteria and Candida to spread up the intestinal tract to inhabit the small intestines and stomach thereby creating nutritional and intestinal disorders.

Polluted internal ecology

A degenerative intestinal flora can become a source of internal pollution. This process of increasing the overall toxicity of the body is commonly termed 'auto-intoxication'. Pollution of the internal ecology is a fundamental cause of symptoms like fatigue, poor concentration, irritability, insomnia, headaches, muscular aches and pains and contributes significantly to the onset of degenerative diseases.

There are many factors contributing to the increase of internal pollution some of which include the Bacteroides bacteria, along with other bacterial groups such as E. Coli which make up the putrefactive bacteria. That is, they are responsible for the rotting decay of matter in the colon. As a result of this decomposition they produce foul odorous gases.

These putrefactive bacteria favour a diet high in animal protein and fats which increases their output of undesirable metabolites. These include substances such as urea, bile salts, phenols, ammonia and other dietary degradation products which are all potentially harmful to the body.

Retention and stagnation

Very few people have three healthy bowel movements per day. The common problems of constipation and irritable bowel syndrome are both a symptom and cause of degenerative intestinal flora. The retention of faeces in the colon for longer than necessary gives the bacteria a greater chance to adapt to the intestinal environment.

This enables them to increase their numbers and consequently the amount of toxic metabolites too. This stagnation of putrefactive waste in the colon also increases the time for toxins and other foreign substances to pass from the intestine into the bloodstream. The prolonged reabsorption of poisonous materials increases the toxic load for the cells when detoxifying organs such as the liver and kidneys are at work.

Other factors which can affect the intestinal permeability include treatments with X-rays, surgical trauma and shock. All these conditions also have a drastic effect on the efficient functioning of the immune system.

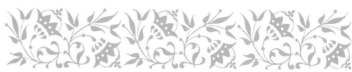

8 Antibiotics to probiotics

Antibiotic use and mis-use

'Bios' means 'life'. Antibiotic therefore means 'anti-life' and they work against life in order to remove the symptoms of infection.

The discovery of antibiotics in the 1930s was a miracle and much suffering has been alleviated through their use in medicine. The extensive use and misuse of antimicrobial drugs has, however, led us to a time in history where we are faced with countless ecological imbalances as a result of this approach to microbial life.

Too much of a supposedly 'good thing' has led to problems such as antibiotic resistance.

Towards probiotics

It is time now to change the recipe and adopt a more positive and constructive philosophy – that of 'pro-life' or 'probiotics'. This means concentrating not on killing the so-called 'bad' microbes, but supporting the many good and beneficial bacteria which are such an integral part of our bodies.

Animals thrive on the addition of live bacteria to their feed. Taking live probiotic supplements is a natural way by which we can personally take responsibility for the imbalances we have created within ourselves through our choice of lifestyle. We need to regain the homeostasis of the bowel. Bifidobacterial probiotics and probiotic tablets have a positive effect on the body because they reduce the internal pollution.

'Bios' means 'life'

The benefits in treating the body with probiotics can be of assistance in the healing of a host of health disorders including:

- Fungal infections e.g. Candida albicans
- Irritable Bowel Syndrome
- Muscular aches and pains
- Allergies
- Skin problems such as eczema, psoriasis and acne
- Cystitis
- Chronic indigestion
- Mouth ulcers
- High cholesterol levels
- Poor immune function
- Gum disease
- Premenstrual tension
- Menopausal problems
- Depression and irritability.

Correcting the balance

Many people who have been on a course of antibiotics complain that the treatment made them feel depressed and exhausted and that they suffered from symptoms of diarrhoea.

When these symptoms occur probiotics in the form of Probiotic-Bifidus powder or tablets should be taken at each meal for at least a month. Probiotic products include:

Bifidobacterial probiotics A quarter of a teaspoon of powder twice daily with food.

Probiotic tablets Two tablets twice daily at meal times.

Live natural yogurt This has a beneficial effect on restoring the environment of the intestine and should be taken daily, two or three tablespoons will be sufficient as a maintenance level.

If you are unwell and have been on a course of antibiotics, increase the amount to four tablespoons, three times a day.

9 Leaky gut syndrome

A condition explained

The lining of the gut is permeable, that is, small particles of food are able to pass through it into the other cells of the body. In a healthy body these 'holes' are small enough to keep contained the molecules which might otherwise cause harm. Besides containing the nutrients we need and which will pass through our permeable gut, food contains a toxic load the body needs to be protected from. This protection is supplied by complex mechanisms which support one another, intestinal secretions, the lining of the intestine and certain white blood cells. It is through this complex system that the digested and important portions of food are able to pass through to the body, the toxins being left out.

However, when the wall of the intestine has been weakened, as is the case with Leaky Gut Syndrome, toxic poisonous substances are released and collected by the lymph nodes which are quite dense in many parts of the body, particularly in the intestinal area as can be seen in the diagram.

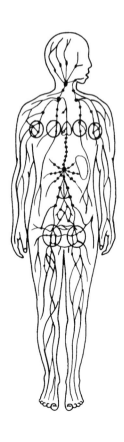

As the lymphatic system flows through the entire human form, lymph nodes are found around major arteries. You can feel raised lymph nodes in the neck when you are suffering from an acute throat infection.

It is so easy to see how a toxic bowel that is leaking destructive substances can circulate its wastes, through the lymphatic system, causing a variety of diseases from arthritis to inflammatory conditions of the kidneys, lungs, brain, and digestive system – to name but a few.

The liver cells serve a very important role by keeping out as much toxic waste as possible, but when it becomes too congested by waste products, alcohol, food additives, etc., its performance becomes compromised.

When there is damage in the intestinal wall due to colitis, diverticulitis, or similar inflammatory states, the number of carcinogens in the liver's function are increased. A toxic condition of the bile is produced which backs up into the pancreatic duct, and this may well be the cause of chronic pancreatic disease.

A damaged intestinal barrier function can also cause disease directly, and it certainly increases the allergic response to foods.

With Leaky Gut Syndrome, numerous health conditions can arise, in particular, chronic inflammatory joint diseases, skin eruptions like acne, psoriasis and dermatitis and many diseases triggered by food allergy, the causes of which originate in the bowel. Amongst the conditions already mentioned, urticaria, eczema and Chronic Fatigue Syndrome can arise from a toxic leaky bowel.

A leaky gut is caused by exposure to substances which damage the lining of the intestine including non-steroidal anti-inflammatory drugs. Other causes are reduced oxygen to the body, as in the case of major surgery, and chemotherapy drugs.

In normal circumstances the lining of the intestine has the fastest production of new cells than any other part of the body; old cells are shed and a new lining is generated every three to six days.

If the gut is damaged the body suffers from inadequate absorption of vital nutrients, and no matter how many vitamins and minerals you add to your diet, absorption will be impossible and the consequence is malnutrition.

The liver of a leaky gut patient works overtime in an attempt to remove oversized food molecules. The over worked liver becomes depleted of certain amino acids: the same condition arises in liver disease caused by excessive intake of alcohol.

Toxicity leads to illness – detoxifying and eliminating returns us to health

Help towards healing

Is it possible to heal a leaky gut? It most certainly is, the body was designed to heal and enjoys being healthy. Many natural substances help repair the mucosal surface of the bowel and help the liver with its vital functions.

Your vitamin and mineral supplements should include all the B vitamins, vitamin A, C and E, zinc and selenium, manganese and magnesium. Glutamine, the amino acid needed for the maintenance of intestinal metabolism, structure and function has been shown to reverse gut abnormalities.

Take essential fatty acids (EFAs) particularly gamma-linolenic acid. Fish oils do help to repair mucosal injury and protect the body from toxins produced in the gut.

However it is recommended that you consider a course of colonic irrigation before you commence on any of the supplements to your diet in order to achieve the maximum benefits. Nature heals well 'on a clean slate' so lets look into the benefits of this very ancient form of healing.

10 Colonic irrigation

An ancient pedigree

Colonic irrigation does not suit everyone, but nevertheless it is becoming a widely used method of cleansing the colon. There is even evidence of colon cleansing by irrigation and herbal preparations being used by the Egyptians, Chinese and Indians for many centuries.

In those days they used large melon shells plus papyrus reeds for the piping: there is mention of the technique in older translations of the Bible. In the early scriptures, which predate the contemporary Bible, the writings of the Essenes also described the technique: 'Seek therefore a large trailing gourd, having a stalk the length of man, take out its inwards and fill it with water from the river which the sun has warmed. Hang it on the branch of a tree and kneel upon the ground. Suffer the end of the stalk of the trailing gourd to enter your hinder parts, that the water may flow through all your bowels.'

There are more accounts of colonics going back to the Egyptian era 1500BC. The Chinese used it long before then; so did Ayurvedic medicine from India, where techniques such as panchakarma included colon cleansing as a part of their routine.

Does it not make sense therefore to accept that the Egyptians, Indians and other cultures who lived a more simple life, living on a natural diet of mostly raw foods, and who enjoyed an environment free of pollution, still felt the need to aid the cleansing of the colon, whereas we now hide away from any discussion regarding the functioning of our bowels?

Herons and other similar birds have been seen in Florida standing by a river filling their beaks with water and injecting the water into their rectums, and then evacuating large quantities of waste matter. They do this without any prior knowledge or training into the benefits of colonic irrigation but with an inborn knowledge of the functioning of the body and how best to preserve it.

Modern practice

Nowadays colonics are performed by an effective series of tubes which are sterilised, then purified water, either fed by gravity or mains fed, enters the colon through a small tube contained in a larger bullet-shaped, comfortably sized speculum which is inserted into the anus and which remains there for the duration of the treatment. There is also a separate exit tube for the removal of faecal waste.

The constant moving action of the warm water breaks up the faecal matter so that the bowel contents are more

The colon can store putrefying toxic material, sometimes for years

easily discharged. The treatment continues for about an hour with constant flushing of the intestine and elimination of the waste.

Any impacted debris which has collected around the walls of the colon are broken down, and after six or more cleansings the patient should feel a renewed energy and many of the aches and pains in the body will have become a thing of the past.

Colonics have given relief to many chronic arthritic sufferers − once the bowel has been cleansed, toxic debris which is residing in the joints are able to be eliminated with ease, liver function is also improved.

Ask a bowel specialist what he thinks about colonic irrigation and he will hold up his hands in dismay at even the thought of such a treatment, and as to the benefits well, are there any?

Ask a bowel specialist 20 years ago whether he considered that diet had a significant factor to play in the cause of bowel cancer, and his reply would be 'absolutely no'.

Ask a bowel specialist the same question today and he would have to agree that statistics tell us that bowel and many other cancers are caused by high fat diets, and that heavy meat eaters are more prone to bowel cancer.

It is even more crazy to have specialists who each deal with a specific function of the human body not understanding the importance of the bowel, when by just reading this book you may well have a better understanding of the bowel and how vital this 25 feet of convoluted tubing is when looking at all the health problems of today.

The benefits of colonic irrigation

These are the simple mechanics of colonic irrigation. Some have likened it to an internal bath, or warm shower.

However, do remember to go to a well qualified practitioner if you decide that a course of colonic irrigation is the way in which you wish to go.

Colonics can help with stress because they encourage us to relax and let go. When we are stressed we tend to hold on tight and this includes the bowel contents as well. Release from the bowel is a true dumping process. Conditions such as diarrhoea, spastic colon, liver sluggishness, halitosis, headache, flatulence, depression, haemorrhoids, skin problems, arthritis, ME, candida, and for those suffering from the distressing eating disorder, anorexia and bulimia, can all benefit.

Diseases of the circulatory system, such as arterial congestion also can have its causes in the digestive system.

The body often dumps its waste matter within the walls of the arteries. Toxins from the colon can stress and weaken the heart, go to the brain and cause confusion and senility; go to the muscles and cause weakness of the body and severe fatigue.

If you decide to consider colonic irrigation to help your health problem, be sure to only eat fruit or steamed vegetables for a couple of days following a treatment.

Colonics can help with stress

Supplements for colon health

To maintain bowel health consider the following supplements to give better colon health:

Linseed Excellent for colon health, a bulking laxative, traditionally used for diverticulosis and other colon diseases. Prevents muscle spasms and reduces inflammation. Contains powerful healing 'omega' oils.

Psyllium husks Soft, cooling, lubricating mucus-clearing, diuretic, absorbs poisons. Traditionally used in dysentery and diarrhoea.

Beet fibre Bulky cellulose fibre for cleansing and stimulating peristalsis.

Slipery Elm Soothing gel protects the intestinal walls from acids and toxins. Traditionally used for ulcers and inflammation.

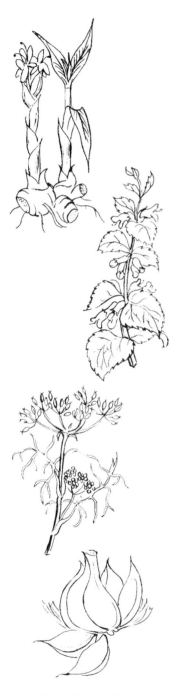

*Ginger, Lemon Balm,
Fennel and Garlic*

Pectin Fruit gel that absorbs toxins, particularly heavy metals and aluminium.

Fennel Seed Calming, warming, containing anethole oil, an antiseptic and local anti-inflammatory. Balances appetite, cramps, colic and flatulence.

Fenugreek Seed Balances appetite and improves assimilation. Makes a warming and soothing bulky gel.

Alfalfa or wheat grass are recommended herbal remedies which cleanse by normalizing the colon's electron balance.

Chlorella and spirulina are additional substances which cleanse the colon.

Fresh garlic is also an excellent antiseptic.

Avoid foods which bind the bowel such as white bread, white sugar, milk and dairy products.

Herbs for the digestive system

Here is a list of herbs which are excellent for helping the digestive system:

Cinnamon A most pleasant and gentle carminative anti-griping, anti-flatulent remedy due to its volatile oils. It helps to prevent bloating, is useful against nausea and due to the tannins it contains has a mild anti-diarrhoeal action.

Yellow Dock This plant acts on the liver and intestines. It is useful for skin conditions where the eliminative and detoxifying functions of the body need stimulating, such as eczema, acne and psoriasis.

Ginger One of the strongest of the aromatic remedies. It contains volatile oils and phenols and has a strong stimulant action on the digestion and circulation. Ginger helps to calm flatulence and colic and is highly recommended for the relief of early morning sickness in pregnancy, or travel sickness.

Lemon Balm A relaxing remedy for the nervous and digestive systems. The pleasant lemony scent comes from the volatile oil in the plant, which also contains bitters and tannins. It is used in the treatment of nervous dyspepsia, indigestion, colic and flatulence.

Meadowsweet This plant is useful for its anti-acidic and anti-inflammatory properties. It contains volatile oil and is rich in minerals. Meadowsweet is recommended for use in problems of acidity, indigestion, heartburn, stomach and duodenal ulcers.

These herbs should be taken as infusions, two or three times a day.

11 Allergy

Increasing toxic loads

We become sensitive to certain substances and foods when the immune system begins to respond to ingested substances as if they were a poison. We frequently crave the food which we are allergic to.

Constant over-reactions by the immune system exhaust it and like a 'tired army' the body gives up and in some cases overacts to almost everything. We then develop a reaction to foods we eat, substances we breath in, substances which we place on our skin. Allergic reactions can cause bloating, sneezing, itchy skin, puffy eyes, irritability, wheezing, headaches, palpitations and fluid retention.

We are prone to allergies more than ever before, as we consume meat which has been produced by cattle fed on artificial foods, antibiotics and hormones, milk from cattle reared on similar foods and drugs. Traces of all these additives get into our systems and eventually into our gut. We breath in more toxins, due to the increase in road and

We frequently crave the food which we are allergic to

air traffic; toxic chemical sprays which are used on our farm land and aerosols which we use in our homes, to name but a few of the irritants which invade our systems. Our immune systems become exhausted as they work overtime in our present day lifestyles.

As our intestinal function becomes congested causing an even heavier toxic load on the immune system, it is hardly surprising that eventually there is a 'straw which breaks the camels back' and the body rebels against the assault.

We then develop our allergies and diseases which are usually treated with a variety of suppressant drugs, yet more toxins invading the body, and more disease as the result.

Good digestion can help

The following are some golden rules to help you to improve your digestion. You should aim to:

Complete digestion is a key to the wellbeing of the intestines and the whole body

- Sit down when eating your meals: eating 'on the run' is disastrous for the digestion.

- Never eat when you are anxious or angry: stressful conditions cause the stomach to 'shut down'.

- Eating smaller amounts more frequently is far better for your stomach and bowels than eating a large meal say, once a day.

- Too much liquid with your food can dilute digestive juices which therefore become less effective.

- Tea and coffee with your meals are bad for your digestion.

- Reduce cows milk to an absolute minimum.

- Avoid cigarette smoke when eating your meals, this can cause havoc with your digestion.

- Only use virgin olive oil for cooking.

- Chew your food thoroughly.

- Avoid the use of aluminium cookware, this metal is known to aggravate digestion.

- Try charcoal tablets to help trapped wind and slippery elm food to assist with digestion generally.

- There is absolutely no doubt that avoiding protein/ starch combinations really does improve digestion.

- Lesions in the thoracic spine can affect the function of your stomach and affect the nerve supply to your intestines. Have some reflexology treatments to aid this or see a well qualified osteopath.

12 Self help to healing

The oldest complementary therapy

Self help is the oldest of all the complementary therapies. Before the advent of free medicine in Britain it was widely practised by people who were too poor to pay for a doctor. In many parts of the world today it is the only medicine available, and regardless of whether you qualify for National Health treatment or are in a private scheme, it is in your best interest to do as much as you can to help yourself.

Drug based therapies are not always the best treatment and, in any case, as has been mentioned before, they only tackle the body part that is affected, never getting to the root cause of the disease which, as you will have learnt now, is at the very base of the disease.

It is in your best interests to do as much as you can to help yourself

Five 'golden rules'

There are five main areas in which you can do much to keep your body in good health.

1. Balance your diet

Firstly, eat a balanced diet, as free as possible from processed high fat and salt content foods. Regard sugar as a 'white poison' since it really does have no food value whatsoever.

The nutritional requirements of the human body can be divided into six groups: proteins, carbohydrates, fats, minerals, vitamins and roughage. We get these things from the food we eat but unfortunately, as has been mentioned previously, so many of our foods have been chemically treated or processed to such an extent that although they look so perfect and attractive from the outside, they have often lost much of their nutritional value.

Crop sprays and fertilisers have left their traces in our foods and these can have an adverse affect on our health and are the cause of so many allergies.

Our bodies consist of countless cells all of which are made of protein and cells require protein for their repair and replacement. Protein is found in meat, fish, eggs, beans, nuts and cheese.

Carbohydrates and fats give us energy and the unit of energy in dietary considerations is the calorie.

We need minerals to help the growth and repair of the body, and calcium to build and maintain our bones and teeth.

Vitamins are substances required in small quantities too, but their absence from our diet can lead to deficiency diseases

Roughage is the name given to indigestible fibres: they simply pass through the body and assist elimination.

The other vital elements are fresh air and water. We must remember that although we are all aware that we breathe through our nose and mouth, our bodies absorb oxygen through the pores, so exposure to the air for the whole body for at least some time during each day is desirable.

Our bodies are composed of between 55 and 70 per cent water. We require an intake of two and a quarter litres per day and we should try to obtain it from the purest source possible. Water today is certainly not as pure as it should be, and in some areas it leaves a lot to be desired.

We should all save hard and get a water filter fitted in our homes, that way our bodies will receive the purest water possible. Tap water should only be used for washing our bodies and general domestic use.

2. Take adequate exercise.
Movement is life. Probably the best exercise is some sport that we enjoy and there are sports to suit all ages. Walking is an excellent form of exercise especially for older people, and has the bonus of getting people out in the fresh air.

3. Avoid stress and anger.
As far as possible, avoid stress and develop a lifestyle that does not stretch your resources up to the limit. Give yourself time to have some pleasurable pastimes.

You will be less stressed if you are engaged in an occupation that uses your talents yet is not beyond capabilities. Ambition is good but to pursue it at the cost of every other relationship is certainly not good for our health.

Are your personal relationships with family, friends, or colleagues as good as they can be? People who 'explode' when frustrations occur, and then forget all about their anger, are doing far more for their health than those who bottle up their feelings. Anger hurts us far more than the person at whom it is directed.

The statement in the Bible, 'Let not the sun go down upon your wrath' is good advice from the health point of view as well as the religious.

You will be less stressed if your occupation uses your talents yet is not beyond capabilities

4. Watch your weight.

Obesity not only puts stress on every organ and function in the body, it also places undue pressure on the skeletal system and bones and joints will wear out faster, if they carry a massive load for many years.

Being overweight makes us susceptible to coronary and renal troubles, diabetes and gallstones.

5. Practise relaxation.

Relaxation can be achieved in various ways. You may wish to join a yoga group and join with yoga relaxation therapies on a regular basis. You may find that you prefer to listen to a relaxing musical tape in the privacy of your own home and concentrate on breathing deeply into your abdomen and letting the body go into a limp state.

Life should not be one endless rush there should be time to 'stand and stare'.

Meditation is as old as religious belief and its main therapeutic value is in combating stress. The principal behind meditation is that you relax and empty your mind of those worries and anxieties that chase each other round and round.

When you have stilled your thoughts in this way you will be led gently into full and effective relaxation.

Since it is difficult to empty ones mind completely, teachers of transcendal meditation and of some other of the Eastern forms suggest that the student chants a mantra; the word 'mantra' simply means thought protection: it is the use of sound, both audible and sometimes inaudible to protect our minds from our thoughts.

If, after taking all precautions to help yourself, you do succumb to some minor ailment, consider self treatment with herbal remedies and reflexology or any other complementary therapy that you feel is right for you.

> There should be time to 'stand and stare'

PART TWO
Reflexology and the link with the intestinal reflexes

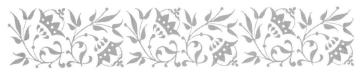

It is not so long ago that few people in this country had heard of acupressure, acupuncture, iridology or reflexology, but today these complementary sciences are being used widely and with great benefits to our general health.

There are reflex points in the colon that react when a body organ is in distress: we can actually map the body by working on the intestinal areas via the feet. Every point along the intestinal tract relates to a specific body part, and a reaction will be experienced by the patient when a deep rotating pressure is applied to these specific body links, if there is inflammation, congestion or tension in that part of the body, or when the body is generally out of balance.

Although I am a great believer in the 'thumb technique', in this instance, as a very deep pressure is needed, you may prefer to use the knuckle of your index finger. Not only does this technique enhance the ability of the Reflexology Practitioner to confirm with even more accuracy which part of the body is in distress but, by applying a rotation to these minute reflex colon points, an even better result can be achieved in all manner of dysfunctions.

In 'Colon Health', Norman Walker states: 'When the operator is giving a colonic irrigation treatment, he or she should **massage the soles of the patient's feet**. This process will help stimulate through the reflexes, the bowel area.'

As an example, if there is congestion in the colon in the area identified as the kidney colon point, it is very likely that the patient will be suffering from congestion in the kidney. This will result in poor elimination of toxic waste, thereby encouraging the formation of kidney stones and kidney infections.

Procedure for accessing the intestinal reflexes in the colon via specific reflex points in the feet.

Before directly accessing the specific points on the feet which link to the intestinal reflexes – as illustrated and explained on the following pages – commence the procedure by applying a massage friction to the inside of both feet with the palm of the hand: this will stimulate circulation to the central nervous system.

Following this, isolate the specific point on the foot/feet that is indicated as relevant to the condition you wish to assist, and apply a deep rotating pressure to it with either the thumb, or knuckle of the index finger, at least 10 times.

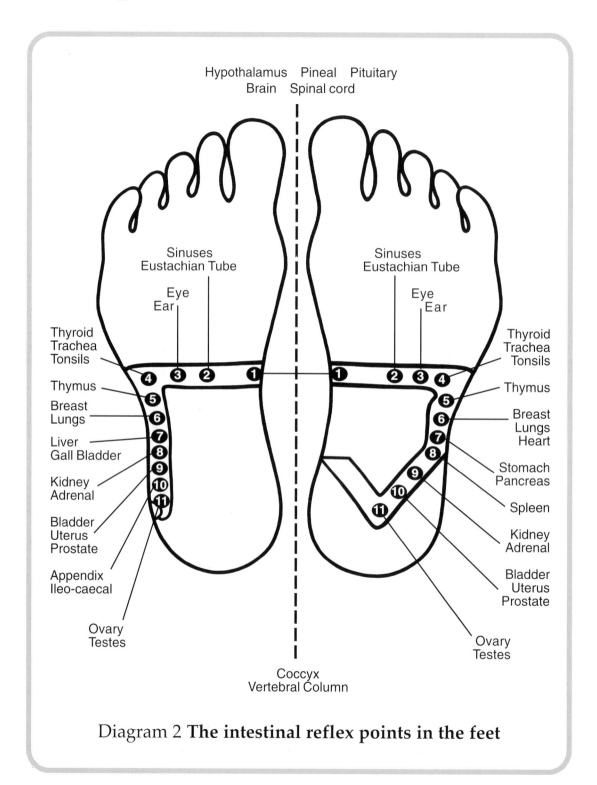

Diagram 2 **The intestinal reflex points in the feet**

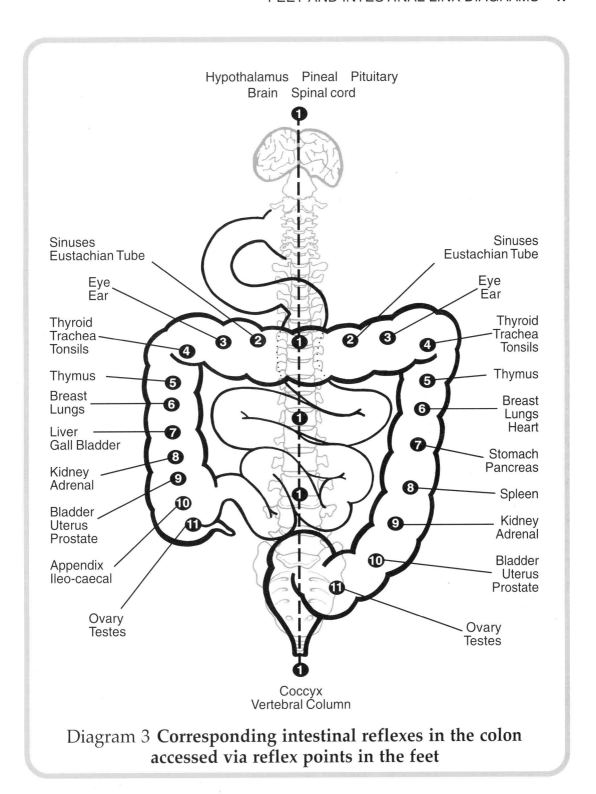

Diagram 3 **Corresponding intestinal reflexes in the colon accessed via reflex points in the feet**

Reflex Point 1

Central – Right Foot and Left Foot

REFLEX POINT 1
Upon isolating this area, apply a deep rotating pressure to this specific point, at least 10 times. **POINT 1** is *the* most important area, as it comprises the pituitary, brain and central nervous system. When assisting with such complaints as hormonal imbalance, premenstrually and also during the menopause, this point would assist in relieving such symptoms as fluid retention, painful breasts and mood swings.

Associated conditions

- **Premenstrual tension**
- **ME - Chronic Fatigue Syndrome**
- **Immune support**

- **Strokes**
- **Infectious diseases affecting the brain**
- **Dementia**
- **Diseases of de-mylineation affecting the spinal cord**
- **Multiple sclerosis**

- **The malfunctioning skeleton**

- **Pituitary, hypothalamus and pineal**
- **The vertebral column, brain and central nervous system**
- **The skeletal system**

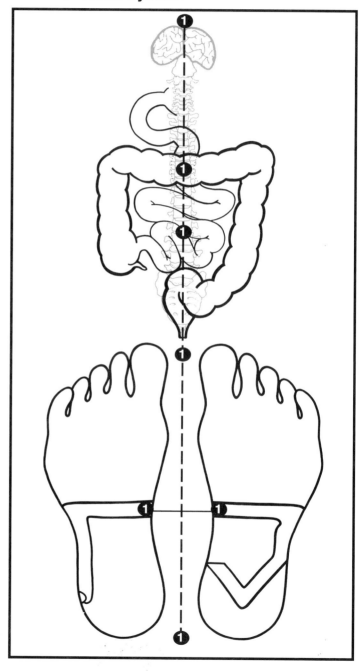

- **Pituitary, hypothalamus and pineal**
- **The vertebral column, brain and central nervous system**
- **The skeletal system**

▨ Premenstrual tension

Most, if not all of your premenstrual discomforts can be alleviated with reflexology and attention to nutrition. This unpleasant condition affects more than 10 million women. It has an effect that goes well beyond mere physical discomfort. It affects the way a woman functions in her job; in school; in coping with her children and her marriage.

Let us look at some facts about oestrogen. As it builds up in the blood stream prior to the onset of menstruation it has an irritating effect on the nervous system. This is the cause for jangled nerves, food binges, irritability, moodiness and other unpleasant characteristics.

It is the job of the liver to prevent the oestrogen build-up. Inside the liver's biochemical factory the B complex vitamins, especially vitamin B6, neutralise oestrogen. The liver cannot do its job without adequate magnesium present in the system. Magnesium combines with the B complex vitamins in an enzyme process that takes on the excess oestrogen. The B vitamins vitalise the magnesium and visa versa.

The first step therefore is to eat a diet high in foods containing magnesium, green vegetables, whole grains such as millet, rice, corn and potatoes. Nuts and seeds are also rich in magnesium but are also high in calories, not recommended therefore if you want to lose weight.

Cut down on sugar. Sugar is a metabolic thief, it robs the body of magnesium and B complex vitamins, both of which are needed to process the sugar for absorption. If you drain the body of magnesium and B complex, you know what happens to the oestrogen levels, they rise!

Sugar also triggers the release of insulin from the pancreas, causing the blood sugar levels to drop. This in

Reflex Point 1

Central – Right Foot and Left Foot

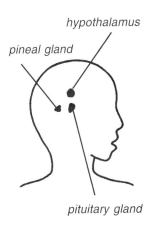

Position of the pineal and pituitary glands and the hypothalamus

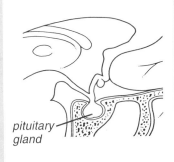

Position of the pituitary gland in fossa

Reflex Point 1

Central – Right Foot and Left Foot

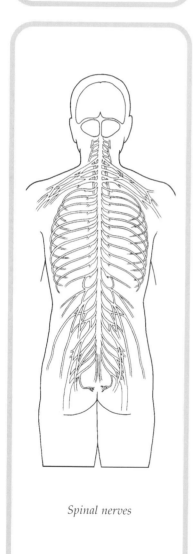

Spinal nerves

- **Pituitary, hypothalamus and pineal**
- **The vertebral column, brain and central nervous system**
- **The skeletal system**

turn can cause tremors, increased appetite, a desire for sweet foods, in particular chocolate, headaches and fatigue. Insulin is a salt retaining compound, this will contribute to water retention and swelling, particularly in the hands, feet and abdominal areas. During the week before the commencement of the period, try cutting down as well on diary products, because calcium blocks the absorption of magnesium, you should take no more than two servings per day. If it is possible to have two reflexology treatments in the fortnight before your period is expected, with dietary and mineral/vitamin support, you could well find that your symptoms soon abate.

■ ME – Chronic Fatigue Syndrome

ME which gives rise to feelings of lethargy, aches and pains in joints, depression and poor immune function, could also respond to working out this point via the intestinal area. ME - frequently referred to as Chronic Fatigue Syndrome is thought to have some link with the Epstein-Barr virus which is a member of the herpes group of viruses. A common aspect of these viruses is their ability to establish a lifelong latent infection after the initial infection. It seems that when the immune system is defective in any way, these viruses can become active for long periods. We therefore also need to work out the **REFLEX POINT 8** which is the link to the spleen and assists our immune function.

Reflexology will assist in enhancing the flow of lymph and improve the blood flow to the spleen and lymphatic tissue. Other methods for stimulating lymphatic flow are by muscle action (exercise and stretching), elevation of extremities, massage, particularly lymphatic drainage massage and hydrotherapy with hot and cold applications.

- **Pituitary, hypothalamus and pineal**
- **The vertebral column, brain and central nervous system**
- **The skeletal system**

▒ Immune support

To achieve good immune function you also need to pay attention to a good diet, high fibre, unprocessed living foods, low fat and moderate consumption of protein. Eight to ten glasses of water per day and a good basic multivitamin and mineral supplement high in the B vitamins, particularly B6, B12 folate and pantothenic acid and the trace minerals: zinc selenium chromium and manganese are essentials. Vitamin C has been found to reduce inflammatory conditions in the body, to have interferon-like and antiviral activity and to enhance white cell destruction of viruses and bacteria.

▒ The brain

The brain resembles a large walnut encased by a strong shell, the shell being the skull. The brain can be divided into three different regions: hindbrain, midbrain and forebrain. Each of these areas perform very different functions. The largest structure in the hindbrain is the cerebellum and this is the area concerned with motor activities. The most important function of our brain is to maintain consciousness.

The brain stem which links the brain with the spinal cord comprises a part of the hindbrain, all of the midbrain and part of the forebrain. It is here in the brain stem that all incoming and outgoing messages come together and cross over, for the left side of the body is governed by the right hand side of the brain and vice versa. The brain really is a very efficient computer that can store information and give an efficient service for the lifespan of its owner. It demands more oxygenated blood than any other part of the body: restrict the oxygen supply and brain cells die rapidly.

Reflex Point 1
Central – Right Foot and Left Foot

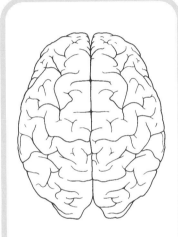

View of brain – superior

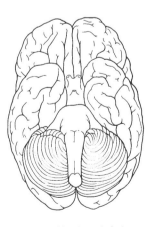

View of brain – inferior

Reflex Point 1

Central – Right Foot and Left Foot

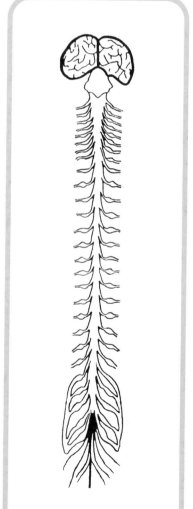

Brain and spinal cord

- **Pituitary, hypothalamus and pineal**
- **The vertebral column, brain and central nervous system**
- **The skeletal system**

▌ Strokes

Many more women than men suffer from this condition, particularly those suffering from diabetes or high blood pressure, and any condition leading to hardening of the arteries – atherosclerosis. Smoking is one of the main causes. Strokes are very common in the over 65 age group and a stroke is a common cause of death.

High blood pressure increases the pressure in the arterial walls. The arteries in the brain are not so strong as in other parts of the body and the weakened wall eventually erupts causing a bleed in the brain. Paralysis of one side of the body is common. Loss of speech, poor co-ordination and dementia are all conditions that can arise following a stroke.

▌ Infectious diseases affecting the brain

Apart from a stroke, other life threatening conditions that can affect brain function are Meningitis or Encephalitis.

Meningitis may be of bacterial or viral origin. Classic symptoms are usually, vomiting, severe head pain and stiffness in the neck. Children are prone to convulsions. Encephalitis is almost invariably induced by a viral infection following mumps, severe attacks of flu and glandular fever.

▌ Dementia

Best known and most feared of the dementias is Alzheimer's disease. This disease can occur at any age but is most common after 50. The incidence of the disease is increasing.

As brain cells are destroyed, particularly in specific areas that are devoted to mental functions, the sufferer becomes

- **Pituitary, hypothalamus and pineal**
- **The vertebral column, brain and central nervous system**
- **The skeletal system**

more and more disabled both mentally and physically.

Clinical trials and recent research have discovered that there is a general reduction in all the neurotransmitting substances that feed the brain. Aluminium levels have been found to be high in sufferers of Alzheimer's, and also very low levels of vitamin B12 have been discovered.

Other less severe dementias, loss of memory and a slowing down in mental reactions is a common feature of the ageing process generally. However, this can be improved by looking into nutritional needs, and many elderly patients have been found to suffer from deficiencies in minerals and vitamins; zinc, selenium and magnesium in particular have been found to be lacking.

We must also take into consideration that many elderly patients are taking prescribed drugs daily, which probably plays a more significant role in the causes of dementia and confusional states than is realised.

▦ Diseases of demylineation affecting the spinal cord

The spinal cord is a roughly cylindrical column of nerve tissues about 40 cm (16 in) long, which runs inside the backbone from the brain to the lumbar vertebrae. It is composed of collections of neurones and bundles of nerve fibres.

The spinal cord has two important functions. Firstly, it acts as a two-way conduction system between the brain and the peripheral nervous system. The second function of the spinal cord is to control simple reflex actions which are achieved by neurones whose fibres extend up and down the cord: these relay messages directly between the sensory and motor neurones.

Reflex Point 1
Central – Right Foot and Left Foot

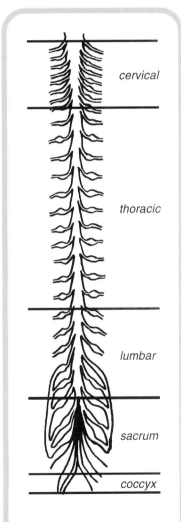

cervical

thoracic

lumbar

sacrum

coccyx

Regions of the spinal cord

Reflex Point 1

Central – Right Foot and Left Foot

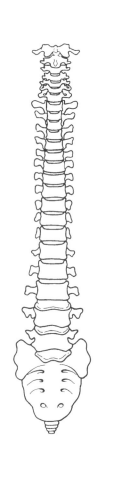

The vertebral column

- **Pituitary, hypothalamus and pineal**
- **The vertebral column, brain and central nervous system**
- **The skeletal system**

If you accidentally touch a live wire, pain receptors in the skin send messages along the sensory fibres to the spinal cord, and you rapidly remove your finger from the stimuli. The same reaction occurs if you put your hand on a hot surface.

■ MS – Multiple sclerosis

This distressing condition is progressive and affects the nervous system. The disease affects the younger generation, particularly in the age range from 20 to 40 years and women are affected more than males.

An interesting feature of the disease is that the country in which you live determines the likelihood of the condition occurring. High risk areas include Canada, New Zealand, Great Britain, Scandinavia and Northern Europe.

The causes are basically unknown although much research has been undertaken to 'unlock the mystery'. Some believe that MS has a viral link; other suggestions are a reaction to certain vaccinations.

Just as certain vaccinations have been known to cause inflammatory conditions of the brain – the whooping cough vaccine was one – there is no reason to suppose why foreign antigens could not be the cause for degeneration of the spinal cord to occur.

It is interesting to note that the incidence of MS is quite low in Japan where consumption of sea foods, seeds and fish oil is high. These foods contain an abundance of polyunsaturated fatty acids, including omega-3 oils. Deficiencies of the omega-3 oils are thought to interfere with lipid elongation and permanently impair formation of normal myeline.

Food allergy, gluten and milk allergy have been linked

- **Pituitary, hypothalamus and pineal**
- **The vertebral column, brain and central nervous system**
- **The skeletal system**

with multiple sclerosis: many patients have benefited from a diet free from wheat and dairy products.

For all dementias and spinal cord deficiency diseases, a daily intake of 40 to 50 grams of polyunsaturated oils is recommended, at least 1 teaspoon of cod liver oil per day and consumption of fish three or more times a week.

Cold-water fish in particular, such as salmon herring and mackerel, are rich in the omega-3 oils. These oils are important in maintaining normal nerve cell function and myeline production.

The skeletal system

The skeleton is a system of struts and levers. It is quite amazing as it twists and bends to permit a wide range of movements unequalled by any man-made machine. The skeletal system is equipped with highly sophisticated shock absorbers, such as the intervertebral discs which cushion each of the bones of the spine.

We are comprised of long bones, short bones, irregular bones and flat bones which are the general framework for the body. Supplemented by cartilage, this softer material covers the ends of many bones.

The bones

Bones support the body's weight, provide the levers needed for movement and protect the soft internal organs. The ribs are rather like the armour of protection to all the vital organs that lie behind this structure.

The bones are moved by muscles which are inserted into them by fibrous structures known as ligaments. All muscles can contract either under voluntary or involuntary control.

Bone is one third water and one of the most biologically

Reflex Point 1

**Central –
Right Foot
and Left Foot**

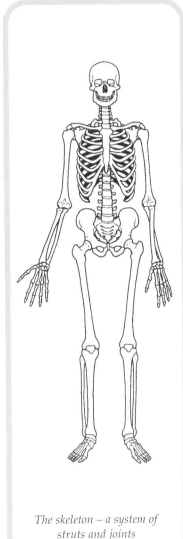

The skeleton – a system of struts and joints

Reflex Point 1

Central – Right Foot and Left Foot

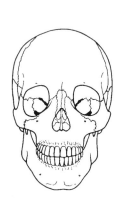

The skull

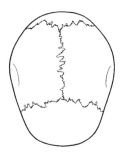

The skull – superior

- **Pituitary, hypothalamus and pineal**
- **The vertebral column, brain and central nervous system**
- **The skeletal system**

active tissues. The body's mineral banks are stored in bone and millions of red blood cells are manufactured every minute in the marrow – the soft core of bone.

There are 206 bones in the normal adult body. The internal structure of bone is made of a tough protein fibre called collagen from the Greek words 'kolla' meaning 'glue' and 'gen' meaning 'forming'.

The calcium and mineral salts provide hardness of bone and strength, making the final structure as tough as reinforced concrete. If the collagen is removed from bone it would crumble; if the salts are removed it becomes as flexible as rubber.

Bone formation and distribution is determined genetically and by the stresses and strains imposed on bone, especially during childhood. Physical activity increases bone volume and density: inactivity results in loss.

■ The skull

The skull, the most protective formation of bone in the body, contains 29 different bones: 14 in the face, 8 in the cranium which are fused together, 2 in the jaw and 3 in each of the ears. The skull is supported by the spine which contains 26 bones called vertebrae.

■ The malfunctioning skeleton

We suffer a variety of aches and pains in our joints and limbs during a lifetime, and the longer we live the more wear and tear will be sustained by our living skeleton.

Replacement parts, which were once a rarity, have now become very common in all orthopaedic departments throughout many countries and include replacement hip

- **Pituitary, hypothalamus and pineal**
- **The vertebral column, brain and central nervous system**
- **The skeletal system**

joints, new knee joints and fusions of discs in the spine.

Spinal curvatures in young children are now a thing of the past, as advancement in surgery allows twisted spines to be straightened by a series of quite remarkable operations.

Sciatica, lumbago, arthritis and all forms of back pain take more people away from their occupations than even the common cold.

We can do much to help ourselves overcome these bodily aches and pains. Sugar, alcohol and high consumption of meat are but a few of the causes. Too much uric acid in the blood stream will often settle in the joints and cause pain. We receive uric acid from an excess of high protein food.

Once again it still all comes down to the bowel. If the bowel and liver are functioning without congestion, uric acid can be eliminated regularly and readily.

Toxic waste will settle in the joints if it has nowhere else to go, so many arthritics have received wonderful relief by tackling their aches, pains and stiffness in a different way. The way forward is colonic irrigation, bowel cleansing herbal preparations and avoidance of the very foods which are not acceptable to the body.

Reflexology treatments will then give longer and better results when the healing energy is not interrupted by an overloaded toxic body.

Reflex Point 1

Central – Right Foot and Left Foot

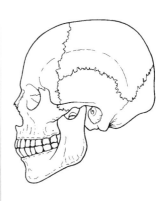

The skull – lateral

Reflex Point 2

Right Foot and Left Foot

REFLEX POINT 2
Upon isolating this area, apply a deep rotating pressure to this specific point, at least 10 times.

Associated conditions

- Sinusitis
- Chronic catarrh
- Hay fever
- Rhinitis

- The sinuses
- The eustachian tubes

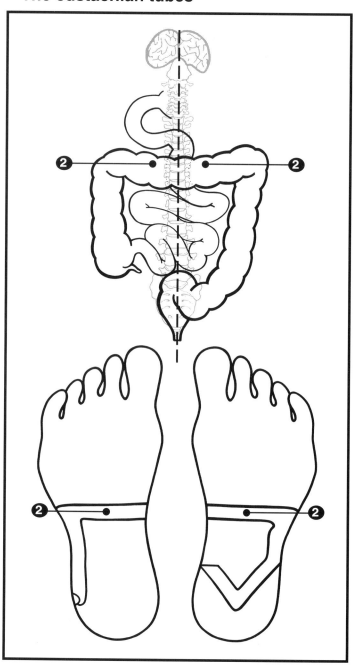

- **The sinuses**
- **The eustachian tubes**

Sinusitis

Sinuses are hollow, fibrous bones within our facial cavities. These bones are hollow in order to lighten the weight of the skull on the neck, to give resonance to our voice and act as drainage of mucus. If the mucus becomes thick and sticky, viruses are encouraged to breed congesting the areas even more and the sinuses then become swollen and inflamed, causing pains in the facial areas.

This results in a streaming cold and sometimes 'flu-like symptoms. If you suffer a fever, it should not be suppressed unless the temperature becomes dangerously high at 40C (104F). While an elevated body temperature may be unpleasant, suppression is thought to suppress a major defence mechanism and prolong the infection. A fever encourages the body to 'burn up' toxic waste.

Sleep and rest are vital factors in encouraging our immune response to function. Our immune system functions better under parasympathetic nervous system control. The parasympathetic system is a part of our autonomic nervous system, which controls and maintains our bodily functioning during sleep.

Consuming plenty of fluids during a cold or attack of sinusitis is vital, as during a cold with a constantly watering nose, we can quite easily become dehydrated. However fluids with a high sugar content, like orange juice or fruit squashes, are not recommended. Sugar greatly reduces the ability of the white blood cells to kill bacteria. Fruit juices and squashes should be greatly diluted.

Vitamin C for general sinus health is recommended and an increased dosage of 500 to 1,000 mg of vitamin C three times a day, during an attack of sinusitis or through a heavy cold, can be taken.

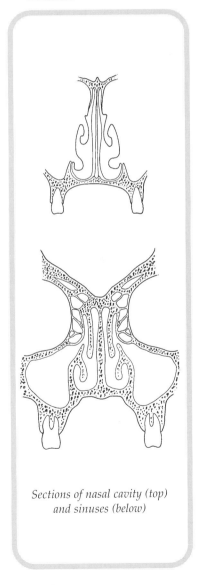

*Sections of nasal cavity (top)
and sinuses (below)*

Reflex Point 3

Right Foot and Left Foot

REFLEX POINT 3
Upon isolating this area, apply a deep rotating pressure to this specific point, at least 10 times.

Associated conditions

- Glaucoma
- Eye strain

- Ear infections
- Glue ear
- Tinnitus
- Vertigo

- **The eyes**
- **The ears**

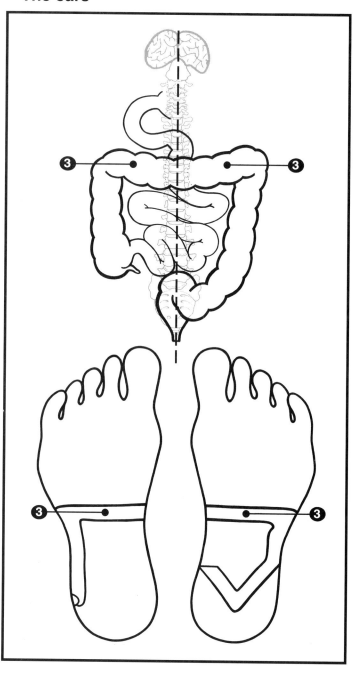

- **The eyes**
- **The ears**

▨ Conditions of the eye

The macula is the portion of the retina of the eye responsible for fine vision. It is located at the centre of the retina. Degeneration of this part of the eye is the leading cause of loss of sight in persons of 55 years and over.

Those with atherosclerosis and hypertension are particularly susceptible. Other conditions affecting the eye are glaucoma, diabetic retinopathy, and any form of emotional stress can drastically affect our visual capacities.

Acute conjunctivitis is commonly due to bacterial infection, the sclera of the eye turning pink or red and becoming painful and swollen. Frequently an infection of this nature arises from infection in the sinuses. Allergic conjunctivitis is associated with hay fever and can cause itching and running eyes accompanied by sneezing.

Ginkgo biloba extract is used primarily to increase the blood supply to the brain, and is recommended in any form of memory loss, senility, etc. Also proven is its role in helping all forms of deterioration of sight. Benefits have also been obtained by increasing consumption of legumes, which are high in sulphur-containing amino acids, yellow vegetables, flavonoid-rich berries, cherries, etc.

▨ Functions of the ear

The ear provides us with the sense of balance as well as our sense of hearing. This complex organ is divided into three parts: the outer ear which gathers sound, the middle ear which is responsible for sound amplification, and the inner ear which converts sound vibrations into electrical impulses transmitted directly to the brain along a pair of nerves which lie side by side. The cochleal nerve is responsible for sound and the vestibular nerve for balance.

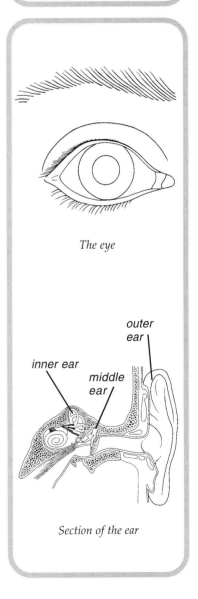

Reflex Point 3
Right Foot and Left Foot

The eye

Section of the ear

Reflex Point 4

Right Foot and Left Foot

REFLEX POINT 4
Upon isolating this area, apply a deep rotating pressure to this specific point, at least 10 times.

Associated conditions

- Hypothyroidism
- Hyperthyroidism

- Tracheitis

- Tonsilitis

- The thyroid gland
- The trachea
- The tonsils

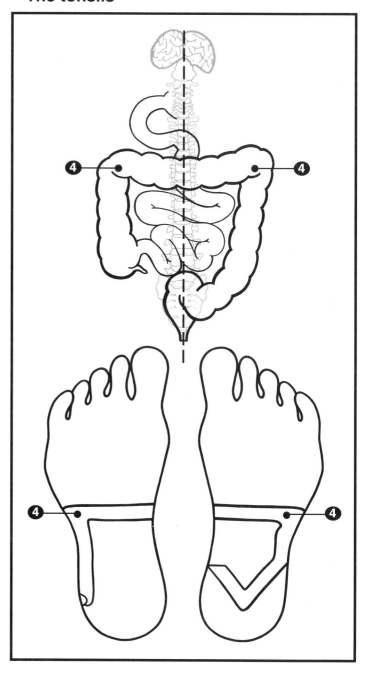

- **The thyroid gland**
- **The trachea**
- **The tonsils**

■ Goitres

The thyroid gland is an 'H' shaped gland which is situated in front of the trachea, and has quite a high failure rate. When this happens the gland will usually enlarge and a large swelling in the front of the throat, called a goitre, will be seen. Goitres may result from insufficient iodine in the diet.

The thyroid is, for some reason, very susceptible to attack by antibodies. Sometime the body produces antibodies which 'attack itself' (auto-immune disease) which may result in an under-production of thyroxine.

■ Hyperthyroidism

Hyperthyroidism or thyrotoxicosis occurs when the thyroid escapes control of the production of TSH from the pituitary. It occurs most frequently in young women who notice increased exhaustion, insomnia, palpitations, weight loss and anxiety. Tremors in the hands are seen: high blood pressure is yet another symptom.

The over-activity of the body affects the peristaltic action of the bowel so diarrhoea is another symptom, and the periods become scanty or sometimes cease altogether.

The increasing amount of energy being expended causes weight loss despite an enlarged appetite: it is as if the body just cannot keep up with the increased metabolic rate. Conventional treatments are anti-thyroid drugs or destruction of the gland with radioactive iodine.

■ Hypothyroidism

Hypothyroidism or myxoedema can be the result of pituitary failure, but is more often caused by damage to the thyroid as the result of drugs, in particular drugs that

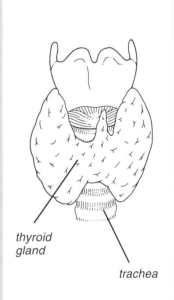

thyroid
gland

trachea

Thyroid gland and trachea

Reflex Point 4
Right Foot and Left Foot

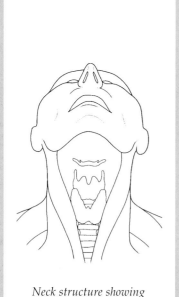

Neck structure showing position of thyroid gland and trachea

- **The thyroid gland**
- **The trachea**
- **The tonsils**

---

treat psychotic disease, such as lithium. Drugs used for certain heart conditions, including cholesterol lowering drugs, can also affect the thyroid.

It is a common condition in menopausal women and leads to weakness and fatigue, rheumatic pains and loss of appetite. All bodily functions slow down. There is apathy, poor memory, aches and pains in the joints, constipation and increasing sensitivity to cold. The hair thins and becomes lifeless. The periods become heavy, and the immune system is affected.

Thyroid disease is epidemic. Approximately one in every 100 people in Britain suffers from an underactive thyroid, and many more people suffer from symptoms of general malaise and do not know the reason why.

■ Thyroid health

It is known that most thyroid conditions are caused by an auto-immune condition – the body actually reacts to its own tissue – but still one of the biggest culprits of all is iodized salt, which is promoted as health-giving all over the Western world.

Pure white salt which has been heated to a considerable level to make it pour with ease, contains no iodine. Iodine is essential for the smooth functioning of the thyroid gland. Salt taken directly from the Salt Mines is rich in iodine. You will find essential iodine in fish, vegetables, milk and meat.

If your thyroid is overactive, try to find ways of removing stress from your life. Take a rest in the afternoon, even 30 minutes can work wonders, and have a full night's sleep every night. Cut out smoking, caffeine and stimulants. Eat small meals frequently, and eat more

- **The thyroid gland**
- **The trachea**
- **The tonsils**

---

calories and protein.

For an under active thyroid, consume iodine containing foods such as kelp and Japanese seaweed. The homoeopathic remedy Iodum Provers can increase levels of circulating thyroid hormones.

Osteopathy can ease symptoms by treating the cervical spine to reduce the muscle spasm and any compressed nerve that may be impeding the blood vessels to the thyroid – another vital area for the reflexologist to work upon when treating deficiencies of the thyroid gland.

Don't forget to take nutrients like selenium, zinc, vitamin E and D, and cold packs applied to the thyroid three times daily can assist in stimulating the function of this vital gland.

▦ Help with asthma

The trachea, a tube which is supported by rings of cartilage and takes air to our lungs, could be a useful point to use when assisting with cases of asthma.

▦ Tonsil function

These small cherry-like glands that are situated on either side of the trachea are lymphatic glands and therefore the first line of defence in the body. They absorb toxins in the form of bacteria and although they swell easily in young children who are more prone to throat infections, they do tend to reduce in size as the child ages and should be retained if at all possible.

A diet free from mucus-making foods which clog these little glands and an increase in vitamin C should help to prevent infections.

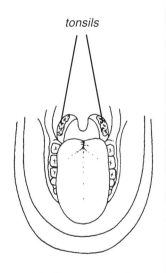

tonsils

Mouth, tongue, teeth and tonsils

Reflex Point 5

Right Foot and Left Foot

REFLEX POINT 5

Upon isolating this area, apply a deep rotating pressure to this specific point, at least 10 times.

Associated conditions

- **Immune system**
- **Cell mediated immunity**

- **The thymus gland**

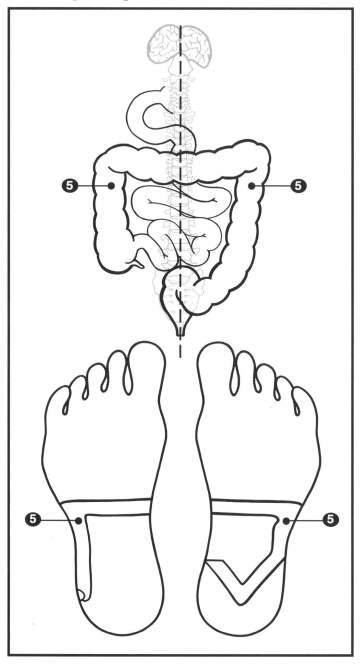

• The thymus gland

▓ Function

The thymus gland is one of the major glands of our immune system. It is composed of two soft pinkish-grey lobes lying just below the thyroid gland and above the heart.

The thymus is responsible for many functions of the immune system, including the production of T lymphocytes, a type of white blood cell responsible for cell mediated immunity. Cell mediated immunity refers to immune mechanisms not controlled by antibodies and is also critical in protecting against all disease.

The thymus gland also produces hormones which regulate many immune functions.

The thymus gland shows maximum development immediately after birth. During the ageing process the thymus undergoes a process of shrinkage and is therefore very sensitive to stress, radiation, infection and chronic illness.

Antioxidants such as vitamin C and E, selenium, zinc and beta carotene can prevent stress on the thymus and enhance the immune function.

Perhaps one of the most widely used herbs for the enhancement of the immune system is echinacea, particularly beneficial to the thymus gland.

Two more herbs which positively affect the thymus gland are liquorice and European mistletoe.

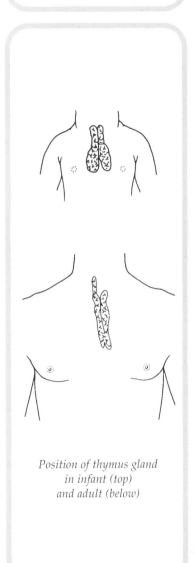

*Position of thymus gland
in infant (top)
and adult (below)*

Reflex Point 6

Right Foot and Left Foot

REFLEX POINT 6
Upon isolating this area, apply a deep rotating pressure to this specific point, at least 10 times.

Associated conditions

- **Fibrocystic breast disease**

- **Bronchitis**

- **Asthma**

- **The breasts**
- **The lungs**

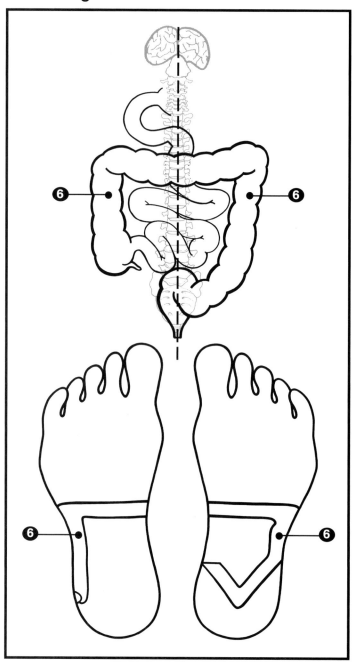

- **The breasts**
- **The lungs**

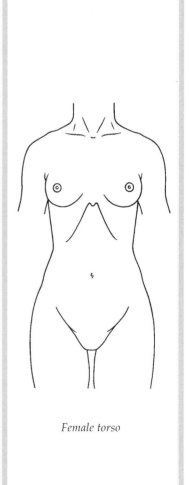

Reflex
Point 6
**Right Foot
and Left Foot**

▨ Fibrocystic breast disease

Fibrocystic breast disease, also known as mastitis is a mildly uncomfortable swelling of the breasts. It is typically cyclic and usually precedes a woman's period. It is the most frequent disease of the breast affecting 20-40 per cent of premenopausal women. It is usually a component of the premenstrual syndrome (PMS) and is considered a risk for breast cancer.

This condition is due to an increased oestrogen-to-progesterone ratio. During the menstrual cycle there is a recurring hormonal stimulation of the breast. As the hormone levels fall after a few days, the breasts return to normal

There is strong evidence supporting an association between fibrocystic breast disease and the consumption of caffeine as found in cola, chocolate, coffee and tea, and many medications. The removal of caffeine from the diet has, in many cases, been the answer to the problem. Vitamin E (600 iu) a day also lowers the elevated levels of the follicle stimulating and luteinizing hormones.

There is a great association between the breast and the bowel which is now being seriously investigated. There is an association between cellular abnormalities in breast fluid and the frequency of bowel movements. Women having fewer than three bowel movements per week have a greater risk of fibrocystic breast disease than women having one movement per day.

The association is probably due to the bacterial flora in the large intestine transforming contents into a variety of toxic metabolites, including carcinogens and mutagens (for more details see Part I).

A simple approach to controlling this disease would

Female torso

Reflex Point 6

Right Foot and Left Foot

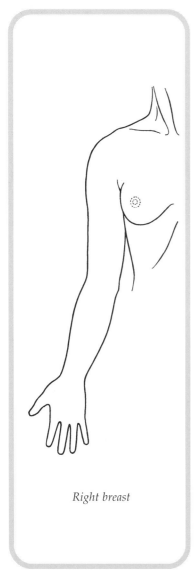

Right breast

- **The breasts**
- **The lungs**

firstly be the removal of caffeine and secondly, cut down drastically on white sugar and increase fluid intake, particularly in the week prior to your period. High fluid increase, in the form of spring water, encourages the body to 'let go' of retained toxins. Take your vitamin B and zinc tablets daily.

▨ Breast cancer

Breast cancer is almost epidemic and it is frightening because it appears to be unavoidable. Every year more and more women are being diagnosed with breast cancer, more than ever before: 186,000 in the US and 33,000 in the UK. It seems that not a day goes by without the announcement of another new avenue to explore, genetic research or better diagnostic treatment. Very few cases of breast cancer have a direct genetic cause.

We *can* help prevent the disease which is a disease of our lifestyle today in the fast track of Western life.

We hear it said that this disease has hereditary links, and most certainly many people seem to have a long family history of cancer recurring. However, habits of families recur also. The way we eat, the type of foods we eat and the type of stresses we are subjected to during our lifetimes are very 'catching'. The way we are conditioned as youngsters to express ourselves, is very 'familial' – habits of a lifetime go on from generation to generation. Maybe environmental and family issues have more powerful links in the development of chronic diseases than we ever imagine.

Cancer requires certain conditions to be present in the body in order for it to develop, just as heart disease is triggered by a combination of high fat foods and a lack of

- **The breasts**
- **The lungs**

---

physical activity, so breast cancer needs a combination of negatives in order to develop.

The evidence is overwhelming in that oestrogen is connected to the development of most breast cancer. Under the influence of oestrogen, cells multiply and swell in preparation for milk production. Oestrogen encourages breast cells to divide more often and more rapidly.

There are two distinct types of breast cancer: the oestrogen-dependent breast cancer and the less common non-oestrogen dependent.

Oestrogen-dependent cancers increased by 130 per cent from the mid 1970s to the mid 1980s. The reason for this is that the average woman is exposed to more oestrogen over a longer period of time than ever before. We have oestrogen in our foods and another important factor to remember is that women live for many years following the menopause.

Pregnancy encourages the breasts to reach full development, until then the cells are more susceptible to abnormal changes, stimulated by hormone production as well as a wide range of cancer causing pollutants. Bearing children helps reduce the risk of breast cancer. Another reason why pregnancy reduces the risk of breast cancer is that during the gestation period, oestrogen supplies are closed while progesterone levels soar. Breast feeding also reduces the risk of cancer. Whilst the baby is suckling, the action stimulates the hypothalamus which then inhibits the release of oestrogen.

By taking the Pill you expose breast tissue to higher amounts of oestrogen.

HRT studies show that this therapy causes eight per cent of postmenopausal cancers and that extended use and high dosages of HRT extend the risk of breast cancer even more.

Reflex Point 6
Right Foot and Left Foot

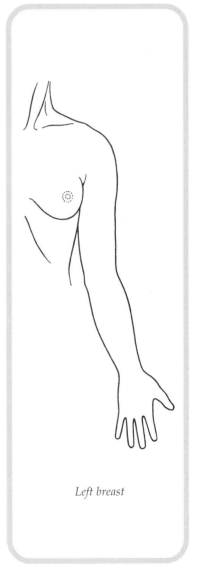

Left breast

Reflex Point 6
Right Foot and Left Foot

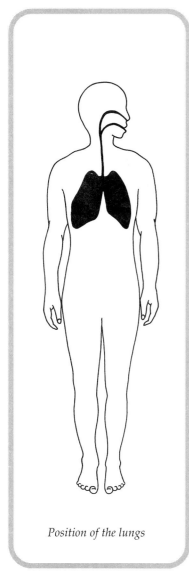

Position of the lungs

- **The breasts**
- **The lungs**

Dietary fat contains a wide range of contaminants, pesticides, industrial pollutants and sex hormones, known to be carcinogenic. Once in the system these pollutants tend to become concentrated in body fat, particularly the breast area. The most dangerous of such chemicals are pesticides, hormones used to bolster meat and dairy production, plastic wrapping and packaging, the dyes used in colouring food and the dyes used to colour your hair: all these have carcinogenic properties.

Aspartamine which is used extensively to sweeten many foods, especially soft drinks, jellies, instant mixes and any foods which advocate their low calorie food value, i.e. the avoidance of sugar, are extremely carcinogenic.

Minimising the risk of breast cancer
- To minimise breast cancer risk, try to maintain a healthy weight. • Keep to a low fat, high fibre diet and cut down on animal fat. • Avoid preserved meat products like sausages, hot dogs and beef burgers. • Limit alcohol which causes oestrogen levels to rise rapidly. • Eat deep-sea fish which are less likely to be troubled by pesticides. • Avoid food packaging, particularly plastic wrapped and canned foods. • Exposure to a microwave, particularly as the microwave is likely to be at breast level, is another contributing factor. Make an effort to stand well away from the microwave while it is in operation. • Stop smoking. Smoking increases the risk of cancer to all parts of the body, not just the throat and the lungs. • Consume unprocessed soya foods, whole grain products, olive oil, garlic and cruciferous vegetables such as cabbage and broccoli. • Increase your exercise. • Avoid as many drugs as you possibly can.

- **The breasts**
- **The lungs**

▨ Problems with the lungs

Lungs are in constant contact with air, yet they are extremely sensitive organs and are affected by pollution, viruses and bacteria more than any other part of the human body.

They are also affected by temperature, which is why air is warmed up or cooled down by our upper respiratory tract before it reaches the lungs.

Delicate layers of mucous membrane line the respiratory tract and any stimulation by pollution causes the membranes to excrete mucus to protect the respiratory system.

Most lung infections proceed from the upper respiratory tract and as the infection and inflammation proceeds into the bronchi, congested passages result which cause irritating coughs and the production of infected sputum. Those most at risk are the very young and the very old.

Chronic bronchitis has become less common since the Clean Air Act of 1956 but it still accounts for 30-40,000 deaths per year, with many more of its victims being severely disabled by respiratory disease leading to breathlessness and eventual heart failure.

Air pollution, dust, cigarette smoke and social factors combine to cause bronchitis. The cilia become damaged so that eventually they cease to evacuate the debris which builds up and leads to irritation of the mucosal cells. These cells become swollen, thus causing the morning cough and further damage to and narrowing of the bronchioles.

In bronchitis and attacks of asthma, the carbon dioxide cannot escape (it is more difficult to exhale than inhale) and so is retained in the blood stream which causes cyanosis resulting in drowsiness and sluggishness.

Reflex Point 6
Right Foot and Left Foot

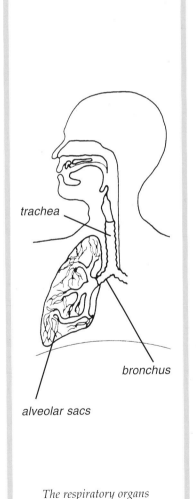

trachea

bronchus

alveolar sacs

The respiratory organs

Reflex Point 6

Right Foot and Left Foot

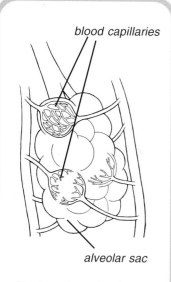

blood capillaries

alveolar sac

Blood supply to alveolar sac

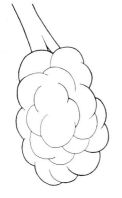

Exterior view of alveolar sac

- ## The breasts
- ## The lungs

Smoking is the main cause of bronchitis and lung cancer. 85 per cent of lung cancer is caused by smoking, the remaining 15 per cent as the result of passive smoking or from those involved in flour mills, asbestos production or other toxic gases which are inhaled frequently.

■ Caring for the lungs

- Obviously, the main assistance in relieving bronchitis would be to avoid pollutants as far as possible. High doses of vitamin C, up to a gram per day, would help to reduce inflammation. • Echinacea, again is such a good immune stimulant in avoiding infection. • Take large quantities of onion juice, a very old fashioned remedy but just marvellous for use as an expectorant. Boil several large onions until they are really soft. Press through a sieve, so that you remove the juice, add some honey to taste and take several times daily. • Garlic also is excellent and fresh garlic should be used in cooking as much as possible. • Avoid all mucus-making foods, i.e. diary products and white sugar. • Only use natural olive oil in cooking.

- **The breasts**
- **The lungs**

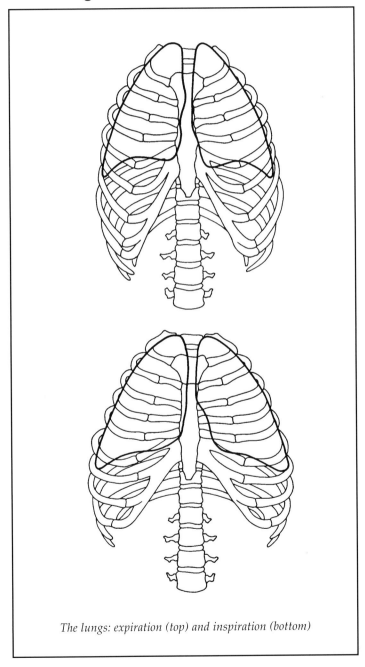

The lungs: expiration (top) and inspiration (bottom)

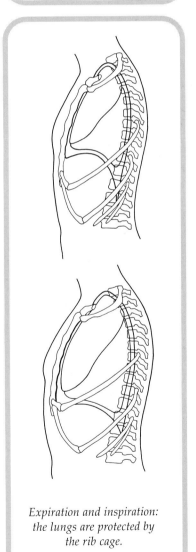

Expiration and inspiration: the lungs are protected by the rib cage.

Reflex Point 6

Left foot only

REFLEX POINT6

Upon isolating this area, apply a deep rotating pressure to this specific point, at least 10 times.

Associated conditions

- **Heart attacks**
- **Angina**
- **Tachycardia**
- **Bradycardia**

- **The heart**

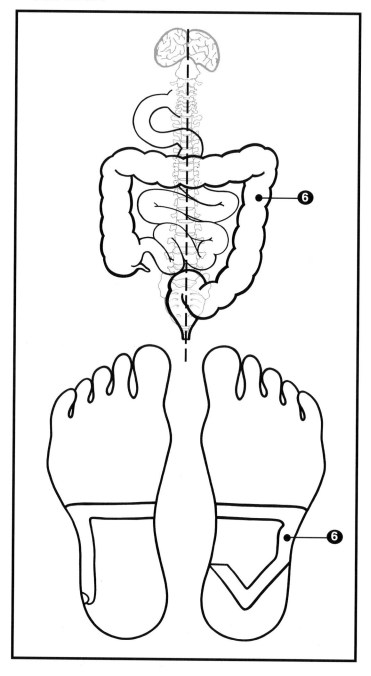

• The heart

▨ An efficient pump

The heart is a muscular pump that works day and night from birth to death. It is an extremely strong tireless muscle, about the size of its owner's fist. However, it can go wrong and unfortunately statistics of death from coronary heart disease are now huge: 170,000 people died in Britain in 1992.

The main function of the heart is to maintain circulation of the blood by pumping it around the body. Its thick muscular walls enclose four chambers: the right and left atria, and the right and left ventricles. The right and left sides of the heart are separated from each other by the septum, and valves ensure that the blood only flows in one direction. The main arteries carry blood from the left ventricle to all parts of the body with each heartbeat: the main veins return blood from the rest of the body to the right atrium, and the two atria contract together and charge up the ventricles with blood. The ventricles then both contract. This ordered series of contractions depends upon a sophisticated electrical timing system.

▨ Blood

Blood is the fuel to the body. Oxygenated blood is needed in order that every cell in the body is nourished, and without this consistent process all functioning fails.

Arteries have thick walls because the blood in them is pumped at force. Veins have valves that stop the blood flowing in the wrong direction and have thinner walls because they do not carry blood at the same force. Veins carry blood containing carbon dioxide and waste products from the body tissues.

Red blood cells carry the oxygen content of our blood:

Reflex Point 6
Left Foot only

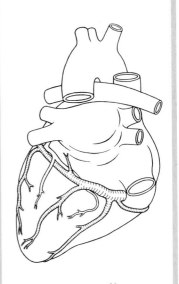

External view of heart

Reflex Point 6
Left Foot only

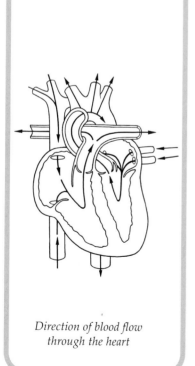

Direction of blood flow through the heart

• The heart

too few and we will suffer anaemia or haemorrhage, and lose a large volume of blood containing red blood cells.

■ Atherosclerosis

The main disease process that thickens and distorts the inner lining of all arteries is called atherosclerosis. In countries in which heart attack is common, such as Great Britain and the USA, early signs of atherosclerosis can be seen in childhood. A heart attack in a man of 50 years of age has its origins in the process of atherosclerosis that began 30 years previously.

The affected areas of the arterial lining are known as atherosclerotic plaques and these enlarge progressively and can bulge into the cavity of the artery. This condition begins when certain white blood cells stick to the lining of the artery, there they collect droplets of fatty substances, particularly cholesterol.

Cholesterol is produced in the liver and is carried in the blood. A high blood cholesterol level is most often due to an excess of LDL – this is the lipid that supplies cholesterol. So when we have a high level of LDL circulating in the blood stream, we run a higher risk of developing atherosclerosis.

By changing your diet so that you replace saturated fats with unsaturated fats your cholesterol level will drop.

■ Heart attack – myocardial infarction

The heart, because it works so tirelessly, needs a generous supply of oxygenated blood and nutrients which are delivered through the coronary arteries. When a branch of a coronary artery becomes blocked, the part of the heart wall that was previously supplied with blood from that

• The heart

branch is damaged, some of it irreversibly, and part of the muscle in the region that has been deprived of oxygen dies (a process called myocardial infarction). In the weeks that follow, the dead muscle is replaced by scar tissue.

Dead muscle cannot contract and therefore the heart becomes a less efficient pump: if severe enough, this can be fatal. Further heart attacks cause more damage and less heart function. The main symptom of heart attack is pain in the chest, arms, throat or jaw.

A more dangerous type of heart attack can be 'painless and silent'. The patient feels ill and weak but as there is no pain to identify the cause, the symptoms are often confused with another type of illness, and the urgency of the situation goes by unnoticed.

▨ Angina

This is more a symptom than an illness, and occurs because the coronary artery is narrowed to the extent that it allows insufficient blood to nourish the heart when there is any exertion. The symptoms are pain in the chest and breathlessness, which improve with rest.

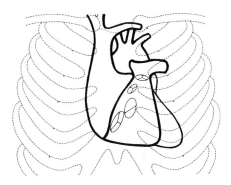

Position of heart within the thorax

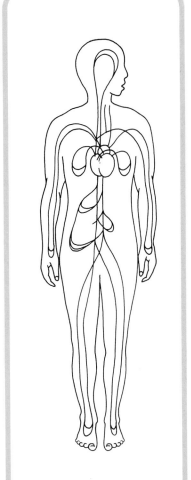

The circulatory system – veins and arteries

Reflex Point 7

Right Foot only

REFLEX POINT 7
Upon isolating this area, apply a deep rotating pressure to this specific point, at least 10 times.

Associated conditions

- **Cirrhosis**
- **Hepatitis**

- **Gall stones**

- **The liver**
- **The gall bladder**

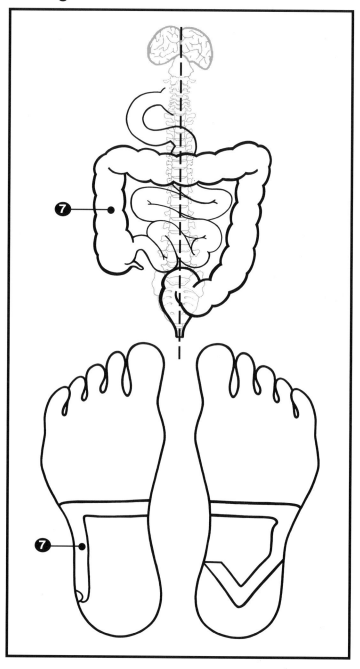

- **The liver**
- **The gall bladder**

▨ Liver function and malfunction

The main function of our liver is to destroy and manufacture. It is the largest gland in the body likened to the efficient working of a large factory where raw materials enter, are converted and finally are despatched or broken down with the aid of innumerable enzymes.

Poor function of the liver will affect all functioning of the body. As the liver is the 'butler to the brain' producing the valuable fuel glycogen which feeds the brain – if it fails, the brain also fails.

The liver is wedge shaped and is on the right side of the body, high up under the ribs. The liver is an extremely vascular organ, blood being supplied by both the hepatic artery, which supplies oxygen, and the portal vein, supplying nutrients.

In cases of heart failure, the reduction in blood flow to the liver causes the liver cells to die.

The reason for any enlargement of the liver is usually hepatitis, cirrhosis or tumour. Apart from cirrhosis of the liver caused by alcoholism, Hepatitis B is another serious condition spread by direct contact of blood, saliva, or semen.

Hepatitis A is spread by the oral-faecal routes: this is the reason why epidemics are common in schools.

We may suffer from jaundice when the small amount of bile which we normally have circulating in our blood is increased to a point where it becomes visible in the sclera of the eyes and the skin. This often happens when there is a blockage in the bile duct, a common cause of which is gall stones.

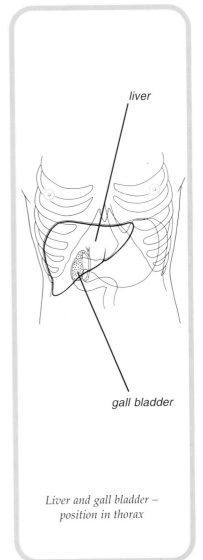

Reflex Point 7
Right Foot only

liver

gall bladder

Liver and gall bladder –
position in thorax

Reflex Point 7

Right Foot only

• **The liver**
• **The gall bladder**

■ Gall stones

Why do so many people get them, particularly women? Oestrogens appear to be a factor, as gallstones are associated with having children, and taking the pill. A highly refined carbohydrate diet is another factor. The chief function of the gall bladder is to concentrate the bile and distribute it through the digestive system. Bile helps to stimulate and lubricate the muscular function of our bowels, called peristalsis; bile also breaks down the fat content in our foods.

■ Biliary colic

This describes the condition where a stone passes down the bile duct causing extreme pain. It is felt mainly in the upper abdomen but can radiate to the lower end of the right scapula. If a stone becomes lodged in the neck of the gall bladder, it leads to pain after meals when the gland contracts.

Symptoms such as nausea, pain and general feelings of malaise accompany this condition, and the removal of the gall bladder usually becomes a necessity to save further occurrences.

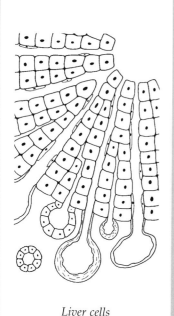

Liver cells

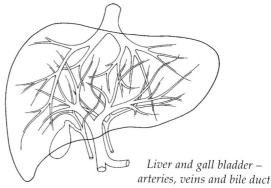

*Liver and gall bladder –
arteries, veins and bile duct*

- **The liver**
- **The gall bladder**

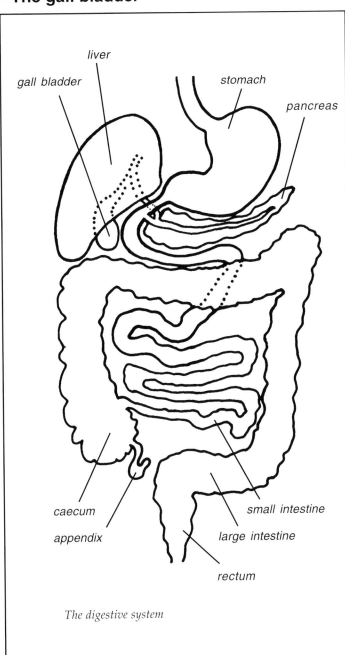

The digestive system

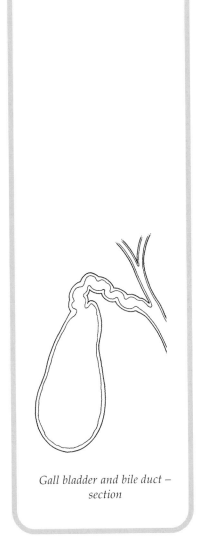

*Gall bladder and bile duct –
section*

Reflex Point 7

Left foot only

REFLEX POINT 7
Upon isolating this area, apply a deep rotating pressure to this specific point, at least 10 times.

Associated conditions

- **Indigestion**
- **Stomach ulceration**

- **Diabetes**
- **Pancreatitis**

- The stomach
- The pancreas

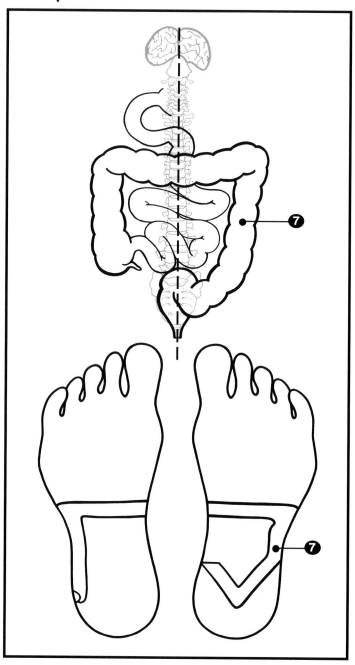

- **The stomach**
- **The pancreas**

▨ Digestion

The stomach is a reversed 'C' shaped muscular sac that lies on the left hand side of the body, in the upper part of the abdomen. It is connected at its upper end to the oesophagus and at its lower end to the duodenum, which is the first part of the small intestine. The pancreas is situated in the curve of the duodenum and releases pancreatic juice into the duodenum via the pancreatic duct to help digest carbohydrates, proteins and fats.

The wall of the stomach consists of a thick muscular layer lined with a special membrane called the epithelium.

Firstly, the stomach acts as a reservoir for food. The lining membrane then produces a special substance which contains acids and enzymes to break down food. In the stomach the food is mixed with digestive juices until it is reduced to a pulp which is then forced into the duodenum. The duodenum measures about 25 cm (10 in).

At the junction between the stomach and the duodenum there is a ring of muscle called the pyloric sphincter, which relaxes from time to time as food is first passed into the duodenum and then into the intestines where further digestion and absorption occurs.

Alkaline juices and hydrochloric acid aid digestion of our food stuffs. Hydrochloric acid in particular breaks down the fat content of our foods.

▨ Stomach ulceration

A high level of stomach acidity causes stomach ulceration, whereas low stomach acidity causes such symptoms as bloating, belching, indigestion, multiple food allergies, weak, peeling and cracked finger nails, acne and iron deficiency: also chronic candida infections.

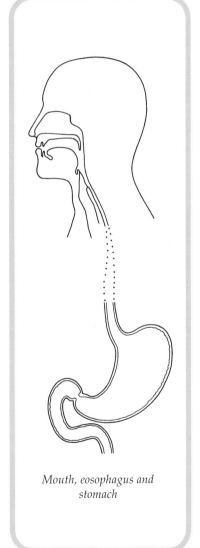

Mouth, eosophagus and stomach

Reflex Point 8

Left Foot only

REFLEX POINT 8
Upon isolating this area, apply a deep rotating pressure to this specific point, at least 10 times.

Associated conditions

- **ME**
- **Arthritis**

• **The spleen**

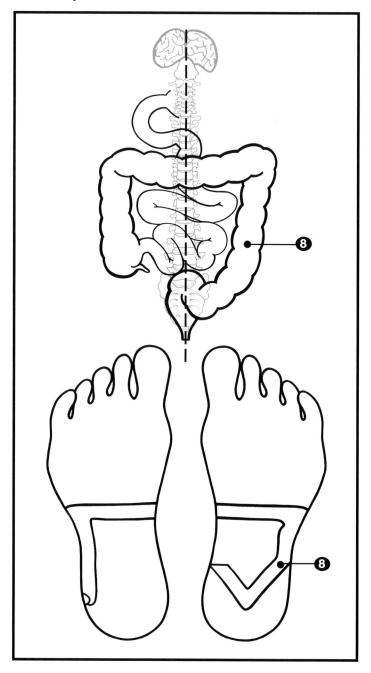

• The spleen

▨ Function of the spleen

The spleen is a major part of the lymphatic system. Its main responsibility is to act as a filter for the blood and to make antibodies. The spleen is about the size of a large dog's pink tongue and lies just below the diaphragm at the top of the left hand side of the abdomen. It is normally about 8 cm (5 in) long and lies along the line of the tenth rib. Its normal weight is about 225 g (half a pound) in adults.

The spleen is supplied with blood via the splenic artery. The arterioles of the spleen are unusual in that they are wrapped in lymphatic tissue as they pass through the pulp of the spleen, this assists the defence mechanism with any abnormal protein in the blood.

The spleen is one of the main filters of the blood, here old worn out blood cells are removed and any abnormal cells are destroyed. It therefore plays an important part in ridding the body of harmful bacteria. It produces antibodies and has the vital responsibility of manufacturing a great deal of the blood of a foetus during gestation.

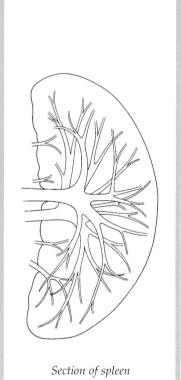

Section of spleen

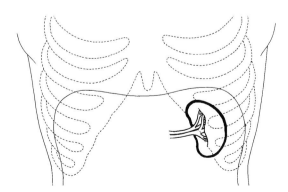

Position of spleen within the body – anterior view

Reflex Point 8

Right Foot only

& Reflex Point 9

Left Foot only

REFLEX POINTS 8 & 9
Upon isolating this area, apply a deep rotating pressure to this specific point, at least 10 times.

Associated conditions

- **Kidney stones**
- **Nephritis**

- **Adrenal exhaustion**
- **Cushing's Syndrome**

- **The kidneys**
- **The adrenal glands**

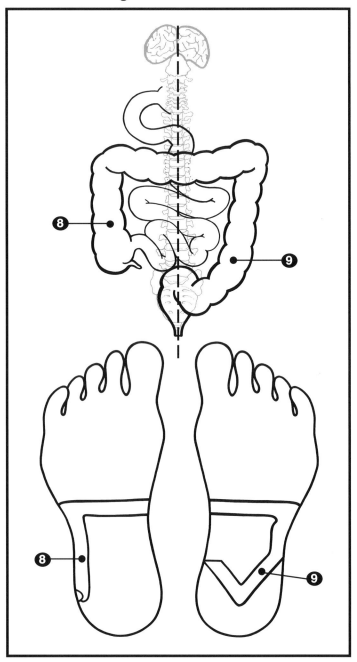

- **The kidneys**
- **The adrenal glands**

▨ Kidney function

These two small bean-shaped organs are organs of excretion and absorption, and lie on the back wall of the abdomen. From the inside of each kidney a tube called the ureter runs down the back of the abdominal cavity and enters the bladder.

The tube leading from the bladder is called the urethra. In women its opening is in front of the vagina and in men at the tip of the penis.

The main function of the kidneys is to maintain a constant fluid and mineral balance in the body.

The Bowman's Capsule, which is the beginning of a tubule, absorbs almost all the filtered water; salt is reabsorbed as well. The reabsorption of water is controlled by a sophisticated system in which a hormone secreted into the blood from the pituitary gland changes the permeability of the tubule. The hormone concerned is the antidiuretic hormone.

Another hormone, aldosterone, secreted by the adrenal glands, is responsible for exchanging sodium salt for potassium salt, which helps to control blood pressure and the balance of salt in the body.

The huge powers of elimination and absorption are quite remarkable from such small, delicate organs. Tiny tubules called nephrons absorb the all-important nutrients which are sent back into the blood stream. 25 per cent of the blood is pumped through our kidneys every minute.

The kidneys are also very responsible for the control of our blood pressure by producing the hormone, renin which the glomerular cells secrete. If these mechanisms go awry hypertension or anaemia can result.

Reflex Point 8
Right Foot only

& Reflex Point 9
Left Foot only

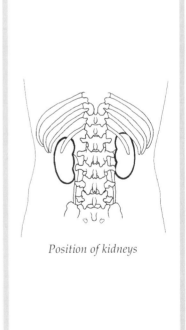

Position of kidneys

Reflex Point 8
Right Foot only

& Reflex Point 9
Left Foot only

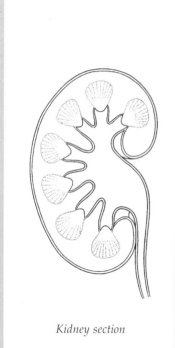

Kidney section

- ## The kidneys
- ## The adrenal glands

▦ Renal failure

When the kidneys fail they no longer are able to secrete urine whose main constituents of water, salt and urea build up in the blood causing oedema, hypertension and uraemia. Urea is an extremely toxic substance which causes total poisoning of the blood and, before the treatment of dialysis became a life saving treatment for those suffering from kidney disease, patients rapidly went into a coma and died.

Renal failure is yet another complication in the case of heart attack, haemorrhage or severe dehydration. This is known as acute renal failure and occurs because the kidney tubules die in large numbers.

Other causes of kidney failure are hypertension, diabetes, polycystic disease and sometimes, renal stones.

▦ The adrenal glands

The adrenals are two small cap-shaped glands. One gland sits on the top of each kidney. Each gland consists of two distinct parts, the inner medulla and the outer covering called the cortex. These parts secrete different hormones, each of which has a different function.

The adrenal glands rarely cease functioning, except in rare circumstances when a benign tumour develops.

The medulla of the adrenal is the part of the gland which secretes adrenaline and its close relation noradrenaline. Together these hormones prepare the body for 'fight or flight' giving the body the ability to perform at its best during times of stress, be it physical or emotional.

The adrenal cortex secretes a series of hormones known as steroids, the most important ones are aldosterone and cortisone.

- ## The kidneys
- ## The adrenal glands

There are three types of steroids: aldosterone, cortisone and the adrenal sex hormones each performing a separate function. The first, known as the salt and water hormone, increases the water retention in the body.

- **Aldosterone**, the principal hormone sends out its chemical messages and instructs the kidneys to reduce the amount of salt being lost in the urine. Salt determines the volume of blood in the circulation which in turn affects the heart's efficiency as a pump.

    When we lose a lot of salt from the body, large quantities of water are lost thereby reducing the volume of blood circulating through the body. Consequently, the heart has to pump harder to send a reduced volume of blood around the body. One can see the dangers here of how the body suffers when dehydration occurs!

- **Cortisone** is responsible for raising the levels of glucose in the blood.

    Glucose is the body's principal fuel and when large amounts are needed in times of stress, cortisone triggers the conversion of protein into glucose. There is only one other hormone in the body that keeps glucose levels down and that is insulin.

    Cortisone is also vital in its capacity to act as an anti-inflammatory and is involved in the functioning of the immune system.

- **Adrenal sex hormones** The final group of hormones produced by the adrenals are known as the adrenal sex hormones, these are secreted by the adrenal medulla and they complement the hormones produced in larger

Reflex Point 8
Right Foot only

& Reflex Point 9
Left Foot only

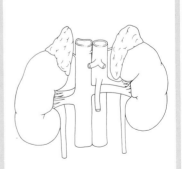

The adrenal glands above the kidneys

Reflex Point 8
Right Foot only

& Reflex Point 9
Left Foot only

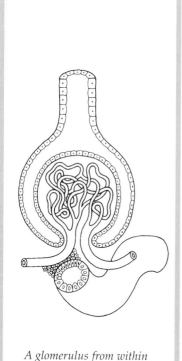

A glomerulus from within the kidney

- ## The kidneys
- ## The adrenal glands

quantities by the gonads – the male and female sex hormones. Testosterone is the principal male sex hormone, also present in women to a lesser degree.

■ Adrenal exhaustion

A common complaint of our twentieth century western living, stimulated by excessive stresses of an emotional nature and encouraged by large quantities of caffeine, food colourings, and excesses of alcohol. Caffeine, in particular, has quite a drastic effect on adrenal function, stimulating its functioning excessively.

More than four cups of coffee a day and you are already over-stimulating your adrenal glands. Adrenal, exhaustion is thought to be the root cause of ME.

■ Cushing's Syndrome

This Syndrome is caused by an excess of circulating steroid hormones in the body and those who have been treated with long term cortisone for asthma, rheumatoid arthritis and multiple sclerosis often fall prey to this condition.

■ Addison's disease

This disease is the opposite condition to Cushing's for here the body has failed to produce hydrocortisone which is required for protection against stress. It may arise from destruction of the adrenal cortex, by a tumour or from TB.

- **The kidneys**
- **The adrenal glands**

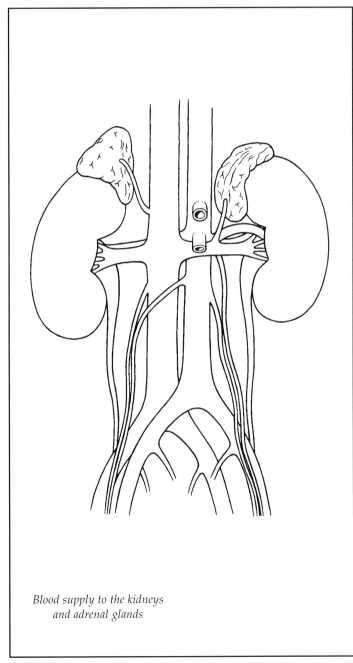

*Blood supply to the kidneys
and adrenal glands*

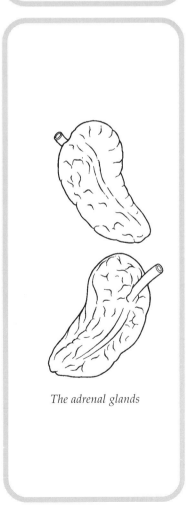

The adrenal glands

Reflex Point 9

Right Foot only

& Reflex Point 10

Left Foot only

REFLEX POINTS 9 & 10

Upon isolating this area, apply a deep rotating pressure to this specific point, at least 10 times.

Associated conditions

- Cystitis

- Endometriosis
- Fibroids

- Prostatitis

- The bladder
- The uterus
- The prostate

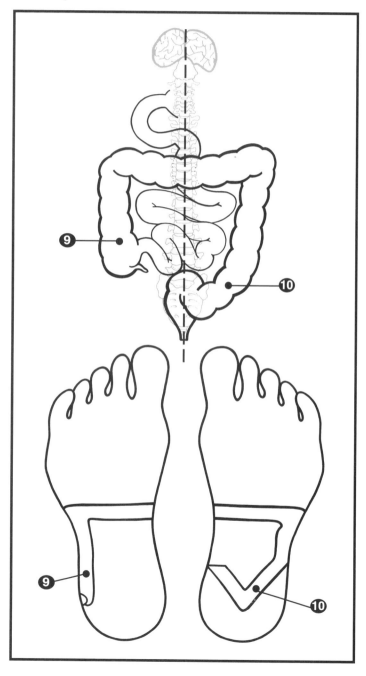

- **The bladder**
- **The uterus**
- **The prostate**

Bladder function

The urinary bladder is a hollow thick-walled muscular organ which lies in the lower part of the pelvic basin between the pubic bones and the rectum.

The bladder is a four sided funnel-shaped sac resembling an upside down pyramid. The base of the bladder provides a surface on which the intestines or, in women, the uterus rests.

The walls of the bladder consist of a number of muscular layers which are capable of stretching, while the bladder fills, and then contracting to empty it. The kidneys pass a nearly continuous trickle of urine down the ureters from the kidneys to its walls. The muscle fibres allow considerable expansion as they adapt to the volume of urine in the bladder. Urine is excreted by the bladder; certain toxic substances such as urea and acids are constantly being formed and these must be eliminated to keep their concentrations in the blood acceptably low. The composition of the urine finally excreted depends on what toxic products the body is producing. Virtually everything found in the urine is present in the blood.

Normally the adult bladder will hold up to half a pint of urine before any discomfort is felt, and emptying occurs before a full pint has been stored. As the bladder fills the stretching of the muscle walls passes signals to the spinal cord.

The uterus

This small pear-shaped sac has remarkable abilities to increase its size to enormous proportions during pregnancy and to shrink back to its normal size which is about equivalent to a plum.

Reflex Point 9
Right Foot only

& Reflex Point 10
Left Foot only

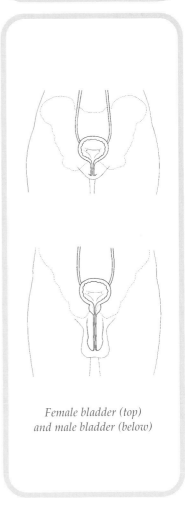

Female bladder (top) and male bladder (below)

Reflex Point 9

Right Foot only

& Reflex Point 10

Left Foot only

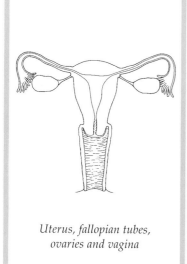

*Uterus, fallopian tubes,
ovaries and vagina*

- **The bladder**
- **The uterus**
- **The prostate**

The uterus is composed of two main parts: the corpus or body of the organ and its cervix or neck.

During the menstrual cycle one egg ripens every month or so between puberty, which marks the onset of a woman's reproductive life, and the menopause which marks the end. Maturation and release of eggs is controlled by hormones from the pituitary gland.

Day 1 While a woman is menstruating the body is busy stimulating the start of the next cyclical change, as egg-bearing follicles begin to ripen, stimulated by FSH (follicle stimulating hormone). The follicular cells produce oestrogen to reinforce the lining of the womb in preparation for pregnancy.

Days 10-12 A surge of oestrogen signals the pituitary gland to produce and release LH (luteinizing hormone), and at this time we may begin to suffer the effects of premenstrual tension, caused by the excess of oestrogen in our blood stream.

Day 13 An increase occurs in LH secretion which causes the follicle to rupture.

Day 14 The ovum is released, ovulation occurs and the ruptured follicle begins its transformation into a yellow body, known as the corpus luteum: this is a rich, proteinous mass in which the ova starts to develop until the placenta forms and takes over the responsibility for the supply of oxygenated blood, rich in all the minerals and nutrients needed to produce a healthy baby.

Days 15-25 The corpus luteum develops further and, in addition to oestrogen, releases another hormone, progesterone. These two sex hormones build up the womb to maximum thickness by producing the endometrial lining in preparation for pregnancy.

- **The bladder**
- **The uterus**
- **The prostate**

■ **Day 26-28** If fertilisation occurs, progesterone and oestrogen from the corpus luteum adapt the uterus to the needs of pregnancy. If the egg is not fertilised, the corpus luteum disintegrates in the last few days of the cycle and the supply of progesterone to the uterus ceases. The lining of the uterus and also the disintegrated corpus luteum is then shed by the menstrual bleeding and a new cycle begins.

■ **Endometriosis**

We hear much about this distressing condition caused by an engorgement of the womb lining, which comes away from the womb and attaches itself to various parts of the body, including the ovary causing ovarian cysts: the bowel and the lining of the pelvic cavity can also be affected.

Endometriosis causes pain, excessive bleeding and in many cases causes infertility.

The use of hormones in our foods today, plus the contraceptive pill which is often taken for many years, is thought to contribute to this growing problem.

Many Naturopaths, and those involved in the principles of the holistic approach to health, feel that when ovulation is suppressed for long periods of time by young women who take the contraceptive pill from as early as 14 years of age or so, the body almost goes into 'overdrive' once the pill is ceased and produces too much uterine lining. It is almost like a rebellious situation!

But we must also take into consideration that a toxic lower bowel can influence the health of the uterus and ovaries, particularly congestion in the sigmoid bend.

Reflex Point 9
Right Foot only

& Reflex Point 10
Left Foot only

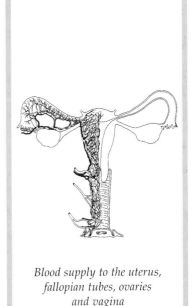

Blood supply to the uterus, fallopian tubes, ovaries and vagina

Reflex Point 9

Right Foot only

& Reflex Point 10

Left Foot only

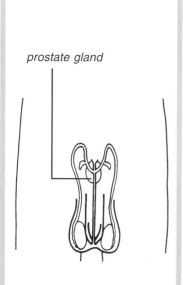

prostate gland

The male reproductive organs showing the position of the prostate gland

- **The bladder**
- **The uterus**
- **The prostate**

▧ Period pains

As the bowel, bladder and uterus are in close proximity to each other, any congestion in the bowel in the form of constipation can play havoc with menstrual pain.

Many a sufferer from years of disabling period pains have been completely freed from discomfort once the health of the bowel has been taken into consideration, a change in diet to enable better elimination and a bowel cleansing programme undertaken.

▧ Problems with the prostate gland

The prostate gland is a walnut-shaped structure found only in males. It is situated at the base of the bladder and surrounds the urethra. This gland produces the fluid that mixes with semen to make up part of the seminal fluid. The seminal fluid is thought to help keep the sperm active so that fertilization can occur more easily.

Owing to its position in the male body, when this gland becomes enlarged or inflamed, normal bladder function can be affected. This is a particular problem in older males and removal of the prostate gland is usually the one sure way of dealing with the situation.

However looking at the problem from a holistic point of view, regular daily doses of zinc plus reflexology treatments have reduced the size of the prostate gland and surgery has then been unnecessary. It is always best to use a gentle approach when treating the body, and use surgery as a last resort.

There has been a dramatic increase in cancer of the prostate gland in recent years.

- **The appendix**
- **The ileo-caecal valve**

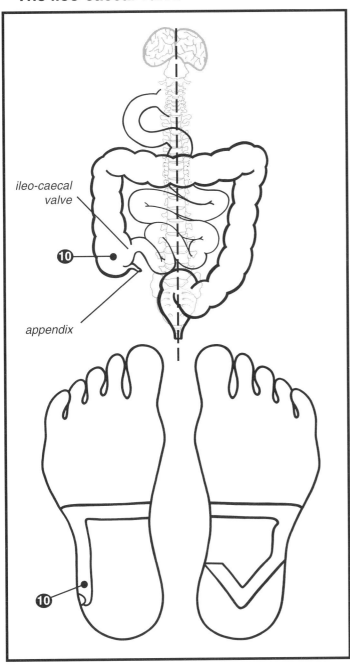

ileo-caecal
valve

10

appendix

10

Reflex Point 10
Right Foot only

REFLEX POINT10
Upon isolating this area, apply a deep rotating pressure to this specific point, at least 10 times.

The ileo-caecal valve is the join of the large and small bowel. When functioning normally, it prevents the back-flow of waste from the large intestines.

The appendix contains lymphatic tissue and aids the health of the bowel.

Reflex Point 11

Right Foot and Left Foot

REFLEX POINT 11

Upon isolating this area, apply a deep rotating pressure to this specific point, at least 10 times.

Associated conditions

- Ovarian cysts

- Testicular cancer

- The ovaries
- The testes

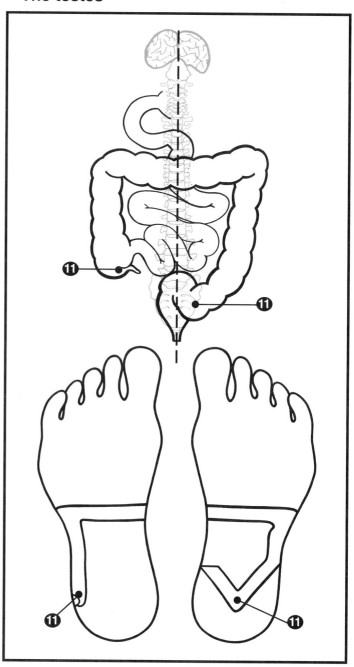

- **The ovaries**
- **The testes**

The ovaries

The ovaries are the parts of the reproductive system which are designed to produce and release ova or egg cells. When the ovum is fertilized by a sperm from a male it triggers the start of a new life.

The ovaries are grey almond-shaped structures about 3 cm long. They reside in the pelvic cavity and lie one on each side of the uterus. Each ovary is held in place by strong elastic ligaments. Just above each ovary is the feathery entrance to the fallopian tube which leads to the uterus.

The ovaries function under the control of the pituitary gland at the base of the brain. The pituitary gland produces a hormone called follicle stimulating hormone (FSH) which travels in the bloodstream to the ovaries. FSH stimulates follicles and ovum development but it also brings about the secretion of the hormone, oestrogen.

Ovarian cysts

Cysts on the ovaries are common in menstruating women and can be relieved and often erupt of their own accord. Reflexology has proved extremely beneficial in treating this condition.

The testes

The normal male has two testes which develop in the embryo. When the testes have formed they gradually move down inside the abdomen so that at the time of birth each testis has found its final position within the scrotum.

The testes are oval structures and at the back of each one is a smaller structure which is rather like a tadpole in shape. This is called the epididymis and collects the sperm from the testes.

Reflex Point 11
Right Foot and Left Foot

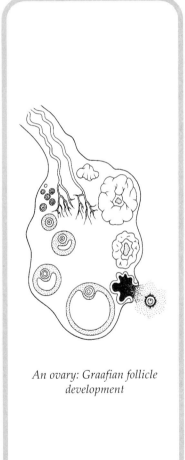

An ovary: Graafian follicle development

Reflex Point 11

Right Foot and Left Foot

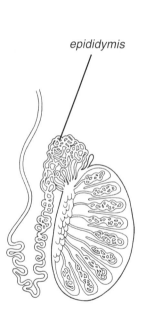

epididymis

Testis and epididymis

• **The ovaries**
• **The testes**

The testes have two functions: the first is to produce sperm and the second function is to produce the male sex hormone, testosterone which activates the male characteristics. These two functions are carried out by different cells within the testes.

We hear too frequently today about the rise in testicular cancer, again this is a Western illness. The causes, as with any other form of cancer, have been dealt with throughout this book, and still the colon has a direct link in the cause of this disease, particularly the sigmoid colon which is in direct proximity to the testes.

■ Infertility

The roots of this increasing problem are again to be found in an increase in the use of hormones, not only in our foods but also in the water we consume due to the fact that hormones are finding their way into water as a result of the elimination of excess hormones in the urine of women who are taking the contraceptive pill or hormone replacement therapy.

Zinc deficiencies are prevalent. We are starved of this mineral which is so vital to the fertility of both men and women. You will have understood by reading this book how a toxic condition of the liver and colon causes the body to be unable to store minerals in sufficient quantities to serve the body's needs.

PART THREE
All about Maria

MARIA'S digestive condition started when she was 13 years old. Maria is very attractive, of slim build with a fine bone structure. She is one of a twin, her sister being much larger and as she says, "She never has any health problems".

The first symptoms that all was not well, was weight loss and feelings of fatigue, which occurred at the same time as she changed senior school. At this time she went on a 'fitness regime' to make a good impression on her new group of school friends. She took up cycling and went on a low fat diet. As her normal weight was only seven and a half stone, her height being 5 ft 2 in, it became very worrying when she dropped to under six stone.

Her mother took her to their GP who diagnosed anorexia, then she started to get lower abdominal pain. She was sent to have a Barium Meal but nothing abnormal was discovered. Maria had not started her periods and as her twin sister commenced hers at the age of 14, there was cause for concern.

Her development seemed to be retarded and so she was referred to a specialist in Endocrinology. She had numerous blood tests, M.R.I. scans, bone density scans – all

of which pointed to the fact that she was not producing sufficient oestrogen.

The next treatment was to commence an oestrogen supplement to induce a menstrual cycle. Her periods commenced but still her weight remained very low.

Maria became depressed. Her doctor recommended a course of antidepressants and she was sent to a counsellor. The antidepressants had no significant benefit on her emotional state and made her very sluggish. She felt that the counselling had little benefit, as she was convinced that her health problems were causing her to be depressed, not the reverse.

Maria remained on the oestrogen supplements until she was 16 at which point blood tests revealed that the oestrogen levels had risen and she was taken off them. However, she was still having the abdominal pains which had started so many years ago, and so 'Irritable Bowel Syndrome' was diagnosed.

In November 1997, when she was 17, Maria was rushed into hospital with a pain that had started in the stomach area and then proceeded downwards into the intestines, on the right side. Appendicitis was diagnosed and the appendix was

removed the same day. Nothing unusual was noted at that time, although some thickening of the lining of the bowel was discovered, a sign of inflammatory bowel disease.

Three weeks after the operation the wound was becoming very painful and it began to swell. Maria then went back to her GP who said that there was an abscess under the wound which would have to be either incised or it would erupt of its own accord.

Maria preferred to let the swelling erupt naturally which it did that night, and she was then left with a gaping area which measured 3 cm x 1 cm. This constantly discharged blood and pus, so she had to wear a dressing over the wound all the time. The erupted area was not particularly painful although it looked angry, so Maria went back to her GP who packed it with gauze. This procedure caused extreme pain, particularly as she had to have this done every day.

The 'packing procedure' continued for two weeks at which point another abscess formed and it erupted again. This routine continued for six months with constant visits to the consultant surgeon who had removed the appendix in the first place.

The area failed to heal so Maria decided to get a second opinion and she was referred to the Royal Free Hospital in London. There she had a Barium Meal, and extensive small bowel Crohn's disease was diagnosed.

Immediate treatment was prescribed with anti-inflammatory drugs and antibiotics. The steroid prednisolone was commenced. These seemed to help the inflammation a little but it did not put the situation into remission. A further drug, azathioprine, was introduced which was an immuno-suppressant. The steroids were ceased. It was said that this treatment would put the 'fire out' which unfortunately it did not do.

At the end of 1998 Maria had a colonoscopy which thankfully showed no disease in the large bowel but a biopsy was taken of the terminal ileum which confirmed the diagnosis of Crohn's disease.

Desperate to find another way

In 1998 Maria consulted me as she was desperate to find another way of improving her health. She was depressed and despondent.

Her life had been drastically affected during this period. She was not well enough to start at university so remained unemployed as she had neither energy or the correct attitude to concentrate on her studies. She remained on her own at home for most of the time as her parents both worked full time: this did not help the situation.

Her examination results suffered as the

result of this illness. She had also been involved in considerable expense in travelling to her repeated hospital appointments in London.

Maria was still taking a considerable concoction of drugs while she was having her reflexology treatments, which affected the very positive results which I feel we could have achieved, had we been able to start treating her 'on a clean slate'.

There was considerable sensitivity in the ileo-caecal valve and also the small intestine. Her liver reflex area too, was extremely sensitive which confirmed to me the changes that had occurred in that organ due to the wide variety of drugs to which she had been subjected.

The reflexes to the spleen also reacted, a sure sign that her immune system had been affected by the prednisolone.

At a further consultation with the professor, surgery was suggested in the form of a resection of part of the small bowel. Maria was horrified at this suggestion and we talked about it during her reflexology treatment and I suggested that she try anything but surgery, which had to be a last resort for a young girl of 18 years of age!

My personal opinion would have been that had surgery been commenced she would have been fitted with a colostomy bag by the time she was 20. As I explained to her, once one part of the bowel is removed, another part will then start becoming diseased as the cause has still not been treated. More surgery will then be performed to remove yet another section of diseased bowel.

A natural approach

What was needed was to get the body into the right state so that it would begin to heal itself.

We talked about homoeopathy to help the general state of her health and Maria consulted a local homoeopath who I knew well and her homoeopathic treatment commenced early in June 1999.

The main benefits that reflexology gave were an immediate release of tension, more confidence in herself and also a general state of well being.

Her back pain which was due to the low bone density, went away and various aches and pains in her joints disappeared also.

Maria felt that the mental benefits were definitely on par with the physical. To-date she is still having treatment with the homoeopath and reflexology with me. She has received more benefits in both these complementary medical therapies in six months than she has in the seven preceding years since her health problem commenced.

The fistula in the appendix area is now healing; it is less raised, much smaller and

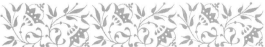

generally not so 'angry'.

Maria now has a regular menstrual cycle not induced with hormonal treatment and has reached a normal weight for her very slight build of eight stone.

The orthodox way

On the orthodox medical approach to her various problems Maria has had the following:

- An operation for the removal of the appendix.
- Countless blood tests.
- Several Barium Meal tests.
- A colonoscopy,
- A liver biopsy,
- Appointments with a counsellor over a six month period.
- Medications: anti-inflammatory drugs, steroids, antibiotics, immuno-suppressants.

Apart from all the distress the patient has suffered, just consider the huge expense to the National Health Service for all the treatments over such a long period.

At the end of seven years of treatment she has added to her list of maladies:

- Reduced bone density
- The effects of steroids, which included a puffy face, red flushed complexion and, as we know, a drastic effect on her hormonal and immune system. And she still had her original problems!

Complementary therapy

It does not take a sledge hammer to crack a nut. Extensive treatments are so often undertaken which are unnecessary. Reflexology and complementary therapies have so far helped in the following ways:

- To-date the fistula above her appendix is healing.
- She now has a normal menstrual cycle without the stimulation of synthetic hormones.
- She has maintained a sensible weight.

Maria's emotional state has improved beyond all expectations: she is happy and confident and commences university this September to study law.

"There always is a simple way to help the body to heal itself".

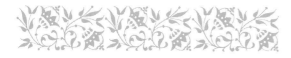

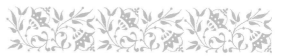

PART FOUR
Understanding stress

WHAT IS STRESS? It is defined as 'any influence that interrupts or disturbs any aspect of the body's normal functioning'.

You may have noticed that whereas one person under stress will develop migraine, another has asthma, someone else gets catarrh, and others suffer from coronary heart disease, ulcers skin disorders or Irritable Bowel Syndrome.

Each of us has a 'weak link'. Overload the link and it will snap. Most of us find that there is one particular part of us that always seems to react when we become over tired, anxious or run down. If you get uncomfortable bowel reactions, your weak point is probably your gut.

What is stressful for one person is perfectly comfortable for another: everyone is different. However, because stress plays such an important part in our lives, we cannot ignore symptoms and just hope that they will go away.

So what is this intangible force that upsets our insides, a force that we cannot touch, see or even describe clearly?

Long ago our ancestors lived in simple caves. They did not have pressures as we have today: the telephone, commuting, traffic jams, demanding jobs, world travel, and trying to bring up young children as well as probably holding down quite a responsible job.

In times of old men were the hunter gatherers and women gave birth and reared their young, and usually breast fed them until they were three years of age and even older sometimes. The child was therefore 'always at the mother's breast' – quite a comforting place to be!

Hunting wild animals to give food to the family was the job of man, and he suffered a considerable form of stress as he went out into the wilderness to search for a wild animal.

His brain would send out messages to his adrenal glands to produce lots of adrenaline. This caused vital changes to take place in his body to give him a better chance of survival. Blood would drain from his skin and digestive system to give more power to his muscles. He would breath faster and deeper to provide that extra energy that would be needed for running and spearing his prey. His pupils would dilate to give him better vision and his blood would thicken and coagulate in case he became wounded.

His blood pressure would rise quite alarmingly as his heart pumped with

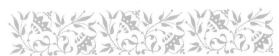
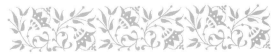

maximum efficiency to give energy for his activities.

In this condition the 'human machine' is in the prime position to fight and survive. Since the dawn of civilisation, and earlier no doubt, mankind has fought a continual battle against physical and mental afflictions. There are, however, many diseases that man has brought on himself either through pure ignorance, blind faith or deliberate misuse of mind and body. One hopes that the improvements in educational facilities, plus the encouragement to help ourselves to maintain better health will assist in eradicating diseases.

Our lives have changed dramatically in the last few million years. Everyday we are exposed to a host of negative influences. These can affect our mood, our attitudes and our general state of mind and then eventually, our health.

We have moved out of caves and, instead, have landed on the moon, invented computers, fax machines, designer clothes and aircraft.

There are endless factors in our life that bother us such as financial problems, pressures of work and family difficulties. The life factors are different but the reactions of our bodies are just the same as our ancestors.

Unfortunately, we do not run for our lives or fight off wild animals; instead, we build up the adrenaline and all the reactions in the body that adrenaline creates. These incidences cause stress.

Some people deal with stress in a positive way, and **stress can be positive**. It can drive us on to achieve and to bring out the very best aspects of our personality. In fact, some people thrive on stress.

For others the slightest pressure or change in lifestyle brings about dramatic changes in mental states, and they become victims to all the stress related illness of today – the hypertension, Irritable Bowel Syndrome, migraine, and so on.

It is long term stresses that lead to physical manifestation of illness. Stress ultimately affects our immune system leaving us wide open to any disease that comes our way. Apart from illness, stressed individuals create tension in the form of excessive perspiration, increased heart rate, rapid and very shallow breathing patterns and insomnia.

The human body was not designed for constant stress and the longer we are exposed to it the less able the body is to deal with it. Should the stress go on for too long, the body eventually becomes exhausted and breaks down. It is not just mental fatigue that we suffer from but a breakdown in our physical health as well.

Cardiovascular disease

Heart disease and all diseases that are responsible for the propulsion of blood

around the body, such as high blood pressure, atherosclerosis, heart attack, angina or a stroke, are almost epidemic in proportion.

We know that dietary habits and smoking contribute to the cause of these diseases but emotional stresses also have a large part to play. It is important to know what can be done to minimise the adverse affects of stress.

Blood vessels are really tubes that transport blood through the body and arteries are blood vessels that carry blood which is pumped from the heart to the different parts of the body. When the vessels dilate with ease, more blood can flow freely and there is less pressure on the vessel wall. When there is constriction, so that the blood flow reduces, more pressure is exerted on the walls of the vessels.

Blood pressure is controlled by several factors. The two minerals, potassium and sodium make up a large part of the equation.

Sodium is linked to constriction of the blood vessels.

Potassium is essential for efficient working of our muscles, and the heart is just a very efficient tireless muscle. Potassium helps dilation of the arteries and relaxation of the muscles surrounding the blood vessels, and also causes a reduction in the retention of sodium and fluid. Both factors lower the blood pressure.

When we are stressed the adrenaline which is released has the effect of constricting the arteries.

These reactions are all fine and produce no damaging effect to the body when the stress is short lived, but a frequent stressed state will certainly have a negative end result as high blood pressure or hypertension is a primary factor in death from heart disease.

Atherosclerosis, or hardening of the arteries, is characterised by the development of fatty plaque in the arteries which progressively narrows the pathway through which the blood can flow. This narrowing creates an enforced pressure on the artery wall and extra effort required from the heart, which will lead to premature death.

Stress has an effect on the immune system. Our immune system protects us from infection. It fights foreign invaders through the production of white blood cells and the activities of the thymus gland.

There are several types of white blood cells. T-Cells are produced in the thymus gland and come in three different forms: T-helper cells which increase immune activity; T-suppressor cells which decrease immune activity; Cytotoxic T-cells which attack infected cells.

T-cells produce interferon which is a substance vital to our immune system.

We produce B-Cells in the bone marrow. These cells manufacture antibodies. Other white blood cells include neutrophils which

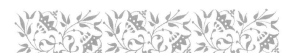
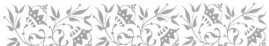

destroy cancer cells and bacteria.

The thymus gland has two functions. It manufactures T-cells essential for regulating immunity and manufactures immune related hormones.

The immune system does an incredible job and works overtime in our lives today due to the toxins which we are bombarded with from the air, and from the increase of all types of pesticides and chemical sprays which are thrust at us from all angles.

When we are stressed or 'tensed up' the body reacts by mobilising and making available resources to the parts of the body where they are needed to deal with the stressful situation. The brain takes priority, then the heart and most important the working muscles in order that you will be able to 'run for your life'.

The result of all this extra energy that is needed in specific parts means that the immune system is deprived of its resources. Stress affects the white blood cells. Corticosteroids, the hormones secreted by the adrenal cortex (such as cortisol) are known to reduce the activity of certain white blood cells that are absolutely vital for resistance to infection.

When secreted during stress, the corticosteroids will generally reduce the resistance to infection as well as to the development of cancer cells. If stress is chronic then the immune system may spend much of the time being underactive. This explains why we are more likely to succumb to disease when going through a particularly difficult period in our life.

If the adrenal glands become exhausted due to chronic stress, the ability for the body to cope with inflammatory states is reduced, which is why we believe stress to be a factor in rheumatoid arthritis, skin diseases and inflammatory bowel disease, to name but a few.

Allergies

Allergic states whether they be related to the skin or asthmatic conditions affecting our respiration are all triggered by stress which constricts the bronchioles in the lungs.

Headaches

Muscles constrict when we are under stress, particularly the muscles in the neck and shoulders. We frequently say, "He or she is a pain in the neck" when describing a stressful situation involving another person.

Dietary elements and stress

Caffeine is a stimulant found in many commonly consumed foods and drinks, including coffee, tea, chocolate and soft drinks such as colas. It is also contained in cough linctus and pain killing, over-the-counter drugs.

Caffeine is relatively harmless when taken in small quantities but is not recommended for those who suffer from chronic stress as

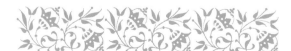

caffeine does cause a rise in the release of adrenaline.

There is also a link between caffeine intake, high blood pressure and raised cholesterol levels. Five or more cups, not mugs, of coffee a day are harmful.

Caffeine has also been linked to causing a reduction to the vital minerals, zinc and iron. Calcium is lost in the urine after caffeine ingestion. We need calcium to aid the efficient functioning of our nervous system. Alcohol in excess creates the same effect as caffeine.

We therefore need to pay attention to the causes of stress, understand the effect chronic stress has on our entire bodily functioning and try to find our own way of 'being kinder to our body'.

You should have learnt much from reading **'Reflexology and the Intestinal Link'** that will help you to understand the vital part our bowel function has to play in the search for a better life quality.

Good health is everything. It is the greatest gift that life can offer us. When we lose our health, everything else we possess becomes of little value.

When we are in a hospital bed with a life threatening condition, whether we are a prince or a pauper the emotional and physical suffering becomes the same.

However we do have choices. We can ignore the warning signals our body gives us and eat wrong foods, drink and smoke, and live in the fast lane and just hope for the best, or open our minds to a better understanding of the body, treat ourselves with respect and make some personal effort to change our lifestyles just as much as we can.

"The choice really is up to you".

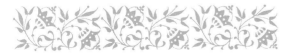
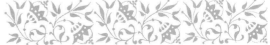

Ann Gillanders' books

**Reflexology,
the Ancient Answer to Modern Ailments**
Published by Ann Gillanders

**No Mean Feat –
Autobiography of Ann Gillanders**
Published by Ann Gillanders

REFLEXOLOGY – The Theory and Practice
Published by Ann Gillanders

**Gateways to Health and Harmony
with Reflexology**
Published by Ann Gillanders

**The Essential Guide to Foot and Hand
Reflexology**
Published by Ann Gillanders

Reflexology and the Intestinal Link
Published by Ann Gillanders

...also available to complement this book:
**The 'Reflexology and the Intestinal Link'
Wall Chart.** Published by Ann Gillanders

REFLEXOLOGY – A Step by Step Guide
Published by Gaia Books

The Family Guide to Reflexology
Published by Gaia Books

.. and a video

**REFLEXOLOGY – The Timeless Art of Self
Healing** *Featuring Ann Gillanders*
Produced by WAVE COMMUNICATIONS Alexandria
Virginia U.S.A.

All the above are available from:
BSR Sales Limited, The Holistic Healing Centre,
92 Sheering Road, Old Harlow, Essex CM17 0JW.
Telephone: 01279 429060
Fax: 01279 445234

Send for our Mail Order Catalogue.